Quick Fixes To Change Your Life

Making Healthy Choices

by

Judy Ann Walz, MSN, RN

Creative Health Services, Inc.
Midland, Georgia

Cover Design: Kathi Dunn, Dunn + Associates, Hayward, Wisconsin
Cover Photo: Dr. Bradley H. Ewald, Beloit, Wisconsin

This publication is designed to provide accurate information in regard to the subject matter covered. It is sold with the understanding that the author and the publisher are not engaged in providing medical care.

Library of Congress Cataloging-in-Publication Data

Walz, Judy Ann, 1945-
    Quick fixes to change your life : making healthy choices /
by Judy Ann Walz.
       p. cm.
    Includes bibliographical references and index.
    ISBN 1-881915-01-8 (pbk.)
    1. Stress management. 2. Mental health. 3. Health. 4. Nutrition.
5. Self-management (Psychology) I. Title.
RA785.W35   1995
613--dc20   94-48587
                                                   CIP

Published by

Creative Health Services, Inc.
7222 Westport Court
Midland, GA U.S.A. 31820-9040
Telephone 0-700-740-6192 or 1-706-568-9006

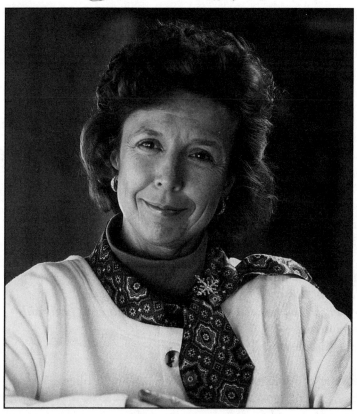

Judy Walz is a community educator on holistic health and a certified psychotherapist. She specializes in self-concept modification and self-valuation, stress management, health consultation, and nutritional counseling. She uses her 20 years of clinical experience in nursing, counseling, and education to teach wellness and self-responsibility. She has a Masters Degree in Nursing and a Masters in Psychology.

Her approach to wellness and health promotion is multifaceted with emphasis on physiology, nutrition, and psychosocial dynamics. She uses humor and a personalized approach to facilitate reaching deep inside and growing beyond the pain and stressors.

In the past 18 years that I've known Judy, I have been the beneficiary of many "quick fixes and healthy choices!" Her extensive training and personal experiences are very evident in the solutions she recommends...
John E. Duerr
Retired President of National Graphics

Attendee comments from Judy Walz's workshops:

Family Support Conference, Kentucky
Please sign your book for me. I enjoyed your workshop in Louisville <u>very much</u>. I know everyone I share your book with will benefit greatly.
BT, Rhode Island

University of Wisconsin-Milwaukee
Excellent presentation, pertinent, positive and mo-tivating....Emphasized the importance of self-care for health promotion.
FM, Wisconsin

Secretary's Seminar Telesis Institute, Alverno College, Wisconsin
Her attitude on life, friends, family, and love is truly refreshing. I left this two-hour workshop wanting and actually needing to hear more....A very inspiring and optimistic speaker....Positive, high-energy, colorful, and mentally exhilarating speaker.

Nursing Seminar, Wisconsin
Judy was great, informative, and fun...I didn't believe only one speaker could hold my interest for six hours and still have me wishing to hear more....Dynamic speaker; her interjected humor is an asset.

*I dedicate this book to my spiritual mentor, the man who has assured me that **angels** do walk here on Mother Earth. May our gifts enrich the lives of others, in love and concern, and enable us to find the right garden in which to grow.*

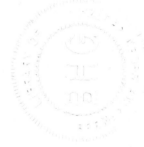

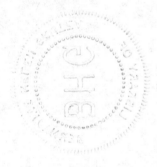

Contents

Foreword

I once encountered an old Zen proverb that said, "When the student is ready, the teacher will appear." How often can we say that the timely occurrence of a special person, a special happening, or even a book has occurred in our lives at such optimal timing that it made all the difference in the world in who and what we are? Such is the unbelievable timing of this superb text. For those of you interested in self-care of a natural and wholesome approach, this text definitely leads the way. Seldom have I found such a complete head to toe assessment addressing everything from spirituality to nutrition all wrapped up in an easy to read format.

In this day of user-friendly computers, it was delightfully refreshing to find a text that allowed me to make my own decisions and chart my own course for achieving health and vitality. You, the reader, will ultimately enjoy the candidness of Ms Walz as she, in her own words and thoughts, conveys what life is like to live in the "not so fast" but healthy lane. The fact that you are reading this note tells me that you are undoubtedly a person interested in the quality of your life, not only tomorrow, but 20, 40, and 100 years from now. Don't put it down. Read it cover to cover and back again. Knowing in your heart and mind that if you follow the "how to" tips of this text, you will undoubtedly become greater than the sum of all your parts. Let Judy Walz and healthy choices become the guiding light in your life so that you, too, can make a difference.

Robert R. Anderson, Doctor of Chiropractic

Introduction

This book is a holistic approach for self-responsible health. As authors flood the literary market with self-help topics, consumers can create more stress in attempting to extract key elements for optimizing their health.

It is my intent to provide a comprehensive compilation of healthy lifestyle alternatives. In this era of *expedience*, decreased health care dollars, and increased exposure to stress and other toxins, this handbook could become a working tool for health (both inside and outside).

Until 12 years ago I worked as a critical care nurse. I felt helpless caring for people in the prime of their life, now entering the hospital with major system failures. For many it was too late for effective life changes. Amid this distress, I made a choice to refocus my commitment to conserving the human resource and my graduate studies reflect that mission. I have a masters degree in psychology and a second masters in nursing focusing on self-care, anger management, and holistic health promotion. I also studied and worked with Dr. Jeffrey Bland in bimolecular nutrition.

For the last ten years I have worked as a community educator, occupational consultant, and psychotherapist emphasizing health promotion, stress reduction, and holistic health. I studied Addiction Interventions to more adeptly provide alternatives and choices before addiction destroys personal integrity.

I carry out each element of this book with my clients. The results are very constructive, positive, self-directed, and promote long-term change for the consumer.

Self-Concept Reprogramming

1

In this book I will break each concept of health into pieces, providing you with alternatives for focused attention and/or personal work. By providing manageable components, it allows you to set priorities for change. I strongly recommend that as one begins any self-exploration, you purchase a spiral notebook to use for a journal. (The spiral is for storing your pen or pencil. You know how they become mobile just when you need them the most). Journaling allows one to externalize discoveries you make about your internal world. If you date your written catharsis, this journal also provides a tangible progress report, positive validation of your assets and growth, especially when you are "stuck," or vulnerable. Ideally, the goal of this book is to invite you to become your own "Very Best Friend." Shall we begin?

Researchers have invested much energy in noncompliance research especially regarding antihypertensive medicines, smoking cessation and substance abuse, elaborate pill counting strategies, patient monitoring, and support groups to assess people's failure to comply with a healthy lifestyle alteration. All these mechanisms are external motivators. In essence, we, as health care providers, have hoped the client would assimilate our definition and value for health. There is substantial evidence that these external, passive-recipient models are not successful in the long-term. Temporary changes occur because the client is the focus of our intentions, or fears reprisal. This fear and control approach has never been compatible with my respect for individuality, and my belief that real change only occurs from the inside out. My basic premise is that unless individuals have a positive sense of self, they will not pursue or value the right to be happy and healthy.

Components of Self-Concept

I must begin a book on healthy choices with a discussion of the components, significance, history, and methods for enhancing a viable, positive self-concept. A person's self-concept is the most important factor affecting human behavior. It is one's *private* self-concept, a map that each person consults to understand oneself, especially during moments of crisis or choice. It gives continuity and consistency to one's personality, and it provides the central core around which *all* other perceptions are organized. Most significant to health is that self-concept is an internal source of self-trust that serves as a guide for personal behavior and relegates other sources of direction to a secondary status. Wouldn't this seem like the most ideal place to begin our quest for health?

The five components of self-concept are self-esteem, personal identity, locus of control, body image, and role performance.

Self-Esteem

Self-esteem is our personal judgment of our worthiness or inner sureness, or lack of the same. It is largely the result of evaluative interactions with others. Early familial experiences play an important role. Our significant others, those

who provide us with a reflective appraisal of our *self*,
continue to nurture or distort our self-esteem. This is the
reference point from which you make decisions regarding
your health state, and when to initiate deliberate action to
achieve a better health state. It provides us with our essence
of lovability. This foundation is laid between the ages of
two to five years.

Personal Identity

Personal identity includes your **core values**, human
aspirations, moral self, and self-consistency. That is, how
we value health, family, community, and how we define
ourselves in these contexts. This component affords us a
sense of congruency and the ability to become "connected,"
or to be socially involved.

Locus of Control

Locus of control is the frame of reference for trust and
serves as a guide for personal behavior. This component
serves as the control-center for decision making, independence, and self-confidence. Your control-center can either
be external or internal or a healthy balance of both.

External control center means that you base your
decisions and actions on the approval or reactions of others
in your life.

Internal control center means that your self-trust
serves as your major guide for personal behavior and
relegates *other* sources of direction to a secondary position.

This is a prime component to deeply embrace, evaluate,
and revise, since predominant internal control creates within you a sense of self-respect, independence, creativity, joy,
and success. If you are predominantly externally controlled,

it results in a chronic sense of defeat/failure, prevailing sadness/depression, increased dependency with potential for co-dependency, and a "no-win" approach to life's challenges. Ideally, we can nurture a balance of both at various stages of our growth and development. However, here is a list of questions to help you explore *where* your control-center is most of the time.

Remember there is no right or wrong answer. Please respond with the most prevalent (70% of the time) response for you now. Consider this a pretest.

Journal

Yes	No	
		1. I am a risk-taker.
		2. I need to discuss my actions with at least three people before I decide.
		3. Once I have all the facts, I can solve most problems and make my own decision.
		4. I tend to buy and wear only clothing that is most popular.
		5. I am usually poised and comfortable among strangers.
		6. I feel good about my personality.
		7. I feel the need to make my parents, family, and spouse proud of me.
		8. I can make my own fashion statement and like being creative and original.
		9. I feel free to express love, anger, joy, resentment, etc.
		10. I need to be connected to a lover to be happy.
		11. I frequently use my children, job, and lover to define who I am.

Yes	No	
		12. I am selfless most of the time.
		13. I am a leader by nature.
		14. I must be happy inside with my decisions.
		15. I am the creator of my own happiness.
		16. I am free to give precedence to my own needs and desires.
		17. I usually feel inferior to others.
		18. I have a driving need to prove my worth and excellence.
		19. I am free to speak up for my own opinions and convictions.
		20. I rarely experience jealousy, envy, or suspicion.
		21. I compare my own talents, possessions, and achievements to others.
		22. I am a "professional people pleaser."
		23. I willingly take responsibility for the consequences of my actions.
		24. I avoid new endeavors due to my fear of failure or mistakes.

Yes	No	
		25. I am often embarrassed by the actions of my family and friends.
		26. I usually judge my self-worth by comparison to others.
		27. I feel uncomfortable, lonely, and isolated when alone.
		28. I base my decisions on the consensus of the group.
		Totals

The closer the totals are to each other the more balanced your internal and external control centers are. The wider the variance of your totals the greater your potential for loss of self to others. This disparity also gives an indication of how easy it would be for you not to have boundaries for defining **self**. Boundaries allow us to know where we begin and end, and where the rights of others begin and end. Boundaries allow us to remain intact in the midst of chaos, because they allow us to take ownership for what issues and behaviors belong to us and which belong to others. This is especially true of emotions like guilt and blame.

Body Image

Body image is another component of self-concept. It is how we perceive our physical attributes, characteristics, and adequacy. This perception will affect one's social interactions, aspirations, and, eventually, self-concept. One's body image is also closely related to whether we base our definition of our physical self on comparison to others (external) or on what we feel is adequate within ourselves (internal). For most of us, the perception of our body image is an area we do not truly accept and cherish until we are in the fourth decade of our life journey (or by age 40). This is a major area of concentration for adolescents because the body image they once knew (as a child) is now undergoing major changes and it can be really scary. Then just when we think our body image is stable, at mid 40s, we deeply recycle the trauma of the adolescent as our body image undergoes another major transition. When we are in the midst of these major transitions, it is imperative that we fortify and nurture the other four components of our self-concept to remain positive and reinforce our real value from the inside.

Role Performance

This is a major area of concern especially as our society is undergoing an industrial and economic crisis. For many persons their job has become their sole source of identity and loss of a job causes a void of self-identity. Also, when one family member becomes ill the roles of every other family member change. One can apply the components of self-concept in defining family strengths and then utilize strategies for fortifying or revising areas of weakness and promote healing and growth of the family system.

In summary, how we value ourselves is central to how we perceive our environment and care for our health. If you regard **self** more positively, there is a greater likelihood that your lifestyle and habits will promote health and optimize wellness. Wellness is not merely the absence of disease, but the harmony of your mind, body, and soul. This harmony requires recognition of these components of **self,** respecting their vitality, and nurturing their growth and resilience. Once we have a positive, viable sense of self, we also perceive events and change as less of a threat to our internal safety. This means less stress in our lives. The stress response is initiated by *how* we perceive an event or situation as a threat to our internal integrity. With a positive sense of self, a crisis becomes an opportunity in work clothes—or, as it translates from the original Chinese word, a dangerous opportunity.

Possessing this internal competency, we can center, gather our resources, identify the problem, explore possible solutions, select alternatives for effective resolution, and then take action to either adapt or accept. We cannot change everything or make all things better. Our focus to conserve and be realistic requires being healthy inside and only then can we make a real difference by "walking our talk" and role modeling congruency and personal responsibility. Health is not external. It can only begin internally by nurturing our own worth, knowing our personal truth, sorting out negative tapes and scripts that we have collected throughout our life, and coming to know our inner truth. Health is really an alliance that we develop with our Creator, to recognize the gifts God has given us, and then to make a commitment to use these gifts optimally in our quest for life as our gifts to our Creator. This cycle is the essence of health.

I will use each of the five components of self-concept and describe strategies that have been very successful for my clients over the last 15 years of clinical practice. Please feel free to try any of them. I promise that they cannot hurt—at least not for long—and that they truly can make a major difference.

Self-Esteem Enhancement

Earlier I mentioned that our self-esteem takes on real form between the ages of two to five years. One could then feel at a loss if these years of one's life were less than ideal. I would like to explore with you strategies that you might use to revise your foundation without razing your entire **self**-structure.

Because our self-esteem is significantly formed in our very early years, often the best way to nurture positive growth is to regress and ask our adult self to reconstruct the dialog for our inner child. My definition of our inner child is the emotional content that largely resides within our chest-navel. It is the physiological area where we **feel** real pain or void when we repeat negative emotions of our childhood. Especially significant are shame and blame, guilt, rejection, and fear of abandonment. Even now, in our adult body, this little child (really our emotional self) vividly recalls the pain as if it were yesterday. The child can repeat the tapes and scripts near-verbatim 30-40 years later. A valid baseline assumption for human behavior is that we repeat affectual reality until we complete the inner work that needs our attention. Affectual reality is the status of our emotional and feeling world. The following w-ire-diagram can serve as a tangible tool to do an autopsy on

behavior and extract the emotional need from which it
initiated.

NEEDS➠ FEELINGS ➠ THOUGHTS ➠ BEHAVIORS

Most of us seem to not move beyond **thoughts** serving
as the motivation for our behavior, or the behavior of our
children. Please remember that **feelings** do not have a
reason—they just are—and they result from a basic human
need (such as security + safety + belonging + love + esteem
= recognition). The only way that we can identify the
underlying feelings and needs is to "turn our head off and
turn our heart on," and to request that our listener do the
same. Then we must not try to **solve** our feelings, but allow
ourselves to verbalize them and internally decide what
inner need is prompting our behavior. Anger is an excellent
way to avoid ever feeling the real primary feelings and to
avoid being vulnerable (childlike). The main motivation for
children's behavior is to avoid pain and to be loved. I really
do not think those motivators change a lot even when we
are in adult bodies. What do you think?

Strategies that have been very successful in reprogramming my clients' self-esteem require journaling to optimize
the identification of **feelings** and **needs.** We never have to
worry about other people exploiting or "putting us down"
because we are self-defeating.

To illustrate this self-destructive tendency just recall for
a moment the last time you made a mistake. Can you recall
what you said to yourself? Something like (perhaps more
intensely punctuated with four letter words) "You stupid
fool, won't you ever learn?" How many hours or days did
this chastising go on? Maybe even four months later, one

can still vividly recall the event and the dialog starts all over.

Now if your best friend made this mistake, what would you say? Something like, "You're only human, anyone could make this mistake. You'll do better next time." We are very generous in our patience for others' humanness and yet very rigid and punitive with our own. Just ponder this thought for a moment—

If you talked to your friends the way you talk to yourself, you wouldn't have any!

All I ask is that you start here with modification and kindness to just become conscious of your self-dialog. Our mind processes on the average of 2,000 words per minute, so the inner dialog that we have fills in when external input slows. Much of our self-dialog is totally unconscious, and it is not until we make this dialog a conscious process that we can revise this destructive habit.

We can only revise habits when we make them conscious reality. It is here that we must first begin, because your self-dialog erodes your self-esteem faster than you can build it. The next time you make a mistake try to constructively assess the event or situation. First set feelings and facts apart, then identify the real issue or problem needing resolution, for example

I shouldn't try to do this task in a hurry.
I need to focus my attention when I do this in the future.

Most accidents and failures occur when we are in a rush, not paying attention, divert our attention, or put our mouth in operation before our brain is in gear.

Does any of this sound familiar? Welcome to the **human race**, and please know that any failure is a lesson in living. If we all were perfect all of the time, there would be little need for another day because there would be nothing more to learn. So, a realistic place to begin revising the "critical tapes" that play in our minds is to set up thought stopping and erase the tape and retape a constructive message.

Quick Fix

Place two fingers on your temple the next time this chastising dialog begins (please note how the idiot verbiage tends to be consistently similar) and say "**STOP**, I won't allow you to speak to me this way." For the first time your adult self will protect your emotional self (the child within) from this punitive reprisal. This process of stopping the tape is best done aloud initially for you to hear your own support. You would not let anyone else talk to you like this, at least not someone that you treasured and wanted to trust. I invite you to try this tape-stopping technique. Each day the critical dialog will decrease. Within three to four days the tapes will disappear, once your unconscious knows that the adult is serving as gatekeeper and filtering out the critical dialog.

The next step is to assess the situation. Identify what you've just constructively learned and replace the chastising dialog with

I'm a student of life and I've just learned another lesson.

As time goes on use problem-solving steps to identify the specific lesson learned. The steps in effective problem solving are as follows (just for review):

Identify the problem or issue

Gather the facts, do some research.

Explore possible solutions (always have more than one choice, success is more likely with contingency plans)

Apply the best solution.

⇓

Evaluate the results. If you're not satisfied, try one of your alternate courses of action

Most of us fail at effective problem solving because we are off and running, trying to resolve the situation before we have identified the problem, not to mention deciding *who* owns the problem. Please remember that we cannot change other people, yet we can change *how* we respond to them. We expend a great deal of energy and hope in attempting to change others or to make them happy. Health and happiness can only begin within ourselves and then we influence others with our centered role-modeling.

For effective long-term change, after your next mistake, use your journal and solitude to sort **feelings** from facts. What hurt you most, i.e., rejection, fear, disappointment, frustration, betrayal? These are just examples. Even joy and love can push our buttons, because positive emotions also may conjure up unmet **needs** and elicit fear. These very positive feelings are something that is foreign to us and we really do not know how to respond. Please be patient with yourself because you are a piece of art still in process.

Self-dialog reminds me of a septic system. We do need to unload some big chunks or have the tank pumped on occasion to avoid backup into our dwelling—which is truly our sense of **self** and how we perceive the world. Many strategies that I will propose are effective methods to remove the septic waste and claim a fresher and healthier view of who we really are. Once you've stopped or at least decreased the frequency of the "critical tapes," replace them with revised ones that nurture your growth.

Revising the tapes requires that you do an inventory of what you do well, what makes you a good person, a good friend, and what makes you unique. Just take five minutes now and write single words, adjectives that describe you best (70 percent of the time—70 percent is a passing grade):

Quick Fix

I am…

I give…

I believe…

I cherish…

Examples may be lovable, honest, tender, forgiving, committed, loyal, humorous, fair, listener, hugger, consistent, growing, and I'm sure this is only the beginning. If this task feels awkward, list five words which best describe the person you love most.

For many of us it is difficult to think of focusing on ourselves, it feels selfish or conceited. Yet we enter relationships hoping that the person will tell us the things that our heart longs to hear—the very things that you know about yourself better than anyone. These validations are the words and reassurance that separate us from others, the deeds and attributes that we offer when no one else is looking. Please remember that it's these very qualities that make us a **masterpiece** and the reason that the Creator gave us each other. Within the very worst of us there is good, in some we just have to look a little harder, but it is there. Each day add a few more discoveries to your list. Invite your family to do the same, that way when you use the words "I love you...," you can add a unique attribute by saying "because ...."

Quick Fix

Using this list of attributes you can now convert them to self-affirmations that will replace the "critical tapes." This is a wonderful gift to give yourself and to anyone you love. Cut place card pieces of colored paper—especially blue, pink, or purple since they are healing colors. Write on these pieces of paper "am honest" or "I love you because your humor makes my heart laugh." Be creative and take the risk. You are telling the truth and you're giving the recipient brief, succinct validation. Make up a stack of them and then fold them into laundry, put them into lunch boxes, suitcases, or jacket pockets. If you are predominantly doing these affirmations for yourself, place them in areas where you are the most vulnerable, for example:

- Inside kitchen cupboards, if meal time is stimulus -over load
- On every mirror in the house so you learn to associate your face with that affirmation
- Use them as book marks
- To the computer terminal, or light switches.

These affirmations are concrete, constructive recognition that you long for others to say to you—and then are disappointed because they have not. These are gifts you can give yourself that enhance your self-esteem, decrease your neediness of others for filling your void, and increase your ability to internalize positive feedback. Many of us have a very difficult time accepting positive input because we have become so addicted to negative dialog; we are even suspicious of positive messages no matter whom they come from.

Personal Identity Nurturance

Strategies for nurturing our personal identity would include the following:

Quick Fix

Define what your epitaph would ideally read.
What do you want your life to stand for?
What will be your gift to this world, what legacy will your life provide?

Perhaps, if we were to consider our epitaph early in adulthood, our life would have more guidance and substance. It is in this process that you can explore just what your ideals, moral standards, and values really are. Much of your personal identity is **how** you operationalize your self-esteem. It also includes how you view your**self** in the context of family and society.

Another strategy that proves effective is to identify your **core values**. These are values that you'd fight to defend, either physically or emotionally. It is these core values that motivate your behavior and elicit internal congruency.

Journal

I value…

List at least five core values that define you as an integral element of society. Examples might include: honor, home, family, freedom, choice, integrity, trust, hope, faith, honesty.

It is important to define core values because when our life or the people in it do not match these values, we feel uneasy, dissonant, and defensive. Until we define these values we do not know what it is we're reacting to; the process of defense is spontaneous. Once the values are clarified, we can make choices that optimize their resilience and viability. We will also be happier when our values are respected. That respect needs to come from within first.

Locus of Control Refinement

In essence, one's locus of control is the primary source of direction and motivation for behavior—the control center. Once we resurrect positive self-esteem, and clarify our values, it will be much easier to pursue our internal directives to maintain congruency of internal and external environments.

The real significance of our control-center is that we need to feel capable of acting on our own behalf to modify life variables, preserving and maintaining our self-respect. The amount and type of stressors that we experience are not as significant as the degree of control that we feel to act or change the situation.

When we rely on external sources for validation and as the cornerstones for our major decisions, there exists a greater tendency for "learned helplessness"—greater stress in living. Depending on external sources for personal worth also increases our tendency to experience chronic disappointment and depression. A baseline assessment and identifying your control-center must begin within **you**. Questions to ask are:

 Journal

1. How often do I say "yes" when I really want to say "no?"

2. How many times a day do I say "I'm sorry?"

3. Do I expend a great deal of energy being a chronic "people pleaser?"

4. Am I passive about my life's course?

If your answer to most of these questions was "yes," then I would propose the following considerations:

1. Identify those persons whose option/values you really respect

2. List those persons whose love/acceptance makes you grow in confidence.

3. Which persons serve as an accurate mirror to reflect the contents of your soul and the qualities that you love most about yourself?

4. What attributes must a person have before you would feel respectful?

Only you can decide if you are allowing outsiders, many of whom you really don't respect in what they've done with their lives or their value-structure, to dictate your life. I encourage you to trust the internal guidance that we all have, be it your intuition or your moral consciousness. We all have the same **scriptwriter**. How we act out our roles in this lifetime relies on internal trust and dialog with our **creator.** The next time you don't really know what to do, I suggest that you only ask for guidance from the Entity who truly knows you from the inside out. Take the time to listen for the reply especially through meditation. Prayer is when we talk to God. Meditation is listening.

Body Image Interventions

Interventions regarding our body image require unlearning much of the idealistic, media-evoked, social- propaganda regarding **how** our body should look. Both men and women have been force-fed subliminal visions of what would make them more sexually appealing, how an ideal body will guarantee them love, and major emphasis on the "package" despite the contents.

What would happen if we focused on the contents being healthy, viable, honest, and happy? Have you ever noticed how some very average looking people have tremendous magnetism and appeal? The way they walk, the joy in their voices, and bright-eyed fervor for living will long outlast the charm of perfect bodies. I am not at all proposing that we neglect or allow our physical body to deteriorate. The health and vitality of our *vehicle* or container are crucial to the *contents*. What I am suggesting is that we put these components of self-concept into proper perspective. We must not allow one area to overshadow the others or to negate all the wealth of potential that we are nurturing in four other areas of personal worth. An effective technique that I have used in my clinical practice is as follows:

Journal

Focus on one area of your body, ideally the most neutral. Avoid beginning this assessment on an area that you are already super critical of, i.e., thighs, waist, or thinning hairline. It is difficult for people to be objective when they are already sensitized to see only the negatives. So, please start with your ankles or your feet and describe the most attractive aspect of your body.

- ► Do your eyes laugh when your mouth smiles?
- ► Is your mouth sculpted?
- ► Does your face take on an entirely different look as it expresses various emotions?
- ► Do you have a lovely smile?
- ► Do you have long, slender, expressive fingers? Do they like to touch?
- ► Is your skin healthy?
- ► No matter body weight, is your body toned and physically fit?
- ► What is attractive about the color of your hair, eyes, skin?

We can only optimize our body image when we start to embrace the positive aspects versus only *see* the negatives. Instead of this external comparative critique, what could happen if we started today to acknowledge something constructive and positive each day. Remember there will always be someone better, yet there will also be someone less fortunate If you have total physical functioning of your body, you are indeed gifted because there are many people who will never know that gift. Instead of commiserating over what you do not have, why not begin celebrating what you do have.

Promoting Role Performance

Strategies for promoting our role performance seem very critical and timely based on the current societal trends. This component is even more critical for males because they have been socialized to believe that their **real** worth is based on their ability to earn money, job status, and possessions. Now when vocations are in transition and undergoing corporate mentality, the patriarchal sense of support and belonging feels more like abandonment or becoming an orphan out on the streets. The impact that this is having on one's sense of loyalty and self-concept is indeed profound.

Of equal significance to me as a clinician, is that this vocational and economic trauma is greatly affecting the increase in domestic violence, suicide, and drug use to avoid the pain of rejection and sense of failure. So if there is an area in which I have a strong interest, especially regarding the survival of a healthy society, it is here. As you might see, the impact of the role performance component will largely be based on how healthy the other four areas are. Perhaps the best way to cope with this area is to maintain positive upkeep on self-esteem, personal identity, body image and locus of control.

Techniques that are effective here are more proactive in nature. It is imperative that you identify tasks, interests, or hobbies for which you have a passion. When you invest yourself in building bird houses, fishing, landscaping, planting, painting buildings or art, dance, music, or singing your soul is fed and you derive joy and sense of purpose.

Become your own salesperson. Apply for a new job every six months, whether you need it or not. In applying for a job every six months, you refine your interviewing skills, request feedback, keep your resume or curriculum vitae updated, and maintain your lateral mobility. I also recommend that you consider two part-time jobs versus one major full-time job. It provides you with an option, variety, decreased dependency, and less vulnerability. We all possess talents that we have not even begun to tap into. What are your areas of greatest aptitudes? Contact your local vocational school and schedule an appointment for a current aptitude test. Meet with a vocational counselor and discover where your aptitudes would have the greatest marketability. Most of us have not taken an aptitude test since we were in high school, if then, so we really have no idea where our skills and talents could be employed at this time in our life.

If your current job has become your sole source of identity, I would strongly encourage you to step back and assess **how** vulnerable that makes you. Where else do you derive your sense of worth? Can you explore other options and/or sources of positive validation?

Another area of concern is how often people use possessions to fill a void for true inner happiness. These folks surround themselves with things. Then they need a larger house to store their things and more security systems to protect their things. They rely on purchasing *things* to elicit joy and internal excitement.

There is a need to balance work with play, for it is when we work the hardest that we need play most to recreate the energy invested in work. Play has no rules, no structure,

and is not competitive, but is unconditional internal rein-
forcement. It is when we forget to play that we become
"crazy -makers." If you never learned to play or forgot
how, ask five-year olds to teach you. They know how to
have a tea party, build sand castles, collect leaves, color and
draw magical pictures, play jacks, build block villages, and
they are so forgiving when you are not perfect. Play allows
nurturing of your self-esteem and healing begins.

Nursing research studies about the effects of one's
self-concept upon the health state have been conducted
after the impact of illness or concurrent with a threat to the
individual's health state. Researchers in the science of
nursing have largely evolved their studies from an illness
model. Therefore, the current research has not reflected an
appraisal of one's self-concept in a state of health. I chose
to consider the benefits of therapeutic intervention to
enhance, nurture, or modify one's self-concept as a preventive measure to retard illness and to enhance coping skills.

In summary, our resilience, ability to remain centered,
make healthy choices, take safe risks, love and maintain
boundaries are all central to our nucleus of self- worth. Our
behavior then becomes *good* for our inner self. Health is
defining what variables, perceptions, and behavior are not
acceptable to us, those that make us comfortable, and those
that the viability of our self-concept will not tolerate.
Learning to make these differentiations and to defuse
potentially harmful situations takes practice and conscious
effort.

Quick Fix

You can best explore safe parameters by using the following affirmations—neutral, limit-setting statements to others when modification is necessary. Start all these exercises within yourself, and then with the next most healthy person you know.

I am not comfortable with this alternative.
I can accept this decision.
I appreciate all your effort at being equitable and
    respecting my concerns.
I find this situation uncomfortable.
I can tolerate this level of ambiguity.

Words like comfortable, accept, and tolerate allow you to honor your values and to protect them using non inflammatory verbiage. They are also words that establish boundaries and affirm your rights as a person, especially for individuals deciding to nurture their self-worth and their internal health. This inner respect will serve as a guide/role model for your external behavior.

As the conclusion to this chapter on self-concept, Please, repeat the following inventory as a posttest.

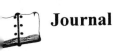

Journal

Yes	No	
	✓	1. I am a risk-taker.
	✓	2. I need to discuss my actions with at least three people before I decide.
✓		3. Once I have all the facts, I can solve most problems and make my own decision.
	✓	4. I tend to buy and wear only clothing that is most popular.
✓		5. I am usually poised and comfortable among strangers.
✓		6. I feel good about my personality.
✓		7. I feel the need to make my parents, family, and spouse proud of me.
✓		8. I can make my own fashion statement and like being creative and original.
✓		9. I feel free to express love, anger, joy, resentment, etc.
	✓	10. I need to be connected to a lover to be happy.
✓		11. I frequently use my children, job, and lover to define who I am.

Yes	No	
✓		12. I am selfless most of the time.
	✓	13. I am a leader by nature.
✓		14. I must be happy inside with my decisions.
✓		15. I am the creator of my own happiness.
	✓	16. I am free to give precedence to my own needs and desires.
	✓	17. I usually feel inferior to others.
	✓	18. I have a driving need to prove my worth and excellence.
✓		19. I am free to speak up for my own opinions and convictions.
✓		20. I rarely experience jealousy, envy, or suspicion.
	✓	21. I compare my own talents, possessions, and achievements to others.
	✓	22. I am a "professional people pleaser."
✓		23. I willingly take responsibility for the consequences of my actions.
	✓	24. I avoid new endeavors due to my fear of failure or mistakes.

Yes	No	
	✓	25. I am often embarrassed by the actions of my family and friends.
	✓	26. I usually judge my self-worth by comparison to others.
✓		27. I feel uncomfortable, lonely, and isolated when alone.
	✓	28. I base my decisions on the consensus of the group.
14	13	**Totals**

32

This time, as you compile your totals, add two points to each of the following items, if you answered YES to them. The items are: 1, 3, 5, 6, 8, 9, 13, 14, 15, 16, 19, 20, and 23.

Now total your answers. If the totals for YES were 22-26, you are more likely to be your own quality-controller, more internally directed, and less likely to experience helplessness or depression as a chronic emotion. Depression is an energy depletor; you feel drained and exhausted. Every one of us can be over-drafted on occasion when our deposits of positive energy are drastically deficient for withdrawals of our resources, very much like a checking account.

My dreams are many
Enjoyed it's true
For I've found myself
A whole new view
Dreams are visions
of what we're due
When leaving to dream
enjoy the view
Although controlling dreams
may be totally new
Faith and will
shall see you through
Think of yourself a student
and know it's true
Death is only graduation
and you control the view.

By Frosty Duckson

Healthy Communication
and
Basic Assertiveness

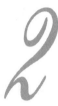 Most stress that we encounter in life is social in nature. Specifically, the source is communication. What a word means to you may not mean the same to me. When the substance of your interaction is very important to you, sort out the key terms and define them before your conversation.

This conserves energy in the decoding process and enhances congruency between the sender and the receiver. It also greatly decreases the stress from erroneous decoding, and, best of all, increases the success of communication.

I will make a commitment to this mission of clarity and success by defining key terms. **Stress** is any demand that requires you to adjust or adapt. You have stress when there is a substantial *imbalance* of the demands and resources you need to respond to or adapt to these demands. It is the common denominator for all adaptive reactions in the body.

Stress management is learning *how* and *when* to center your energies. It means to *act* on your environment before it acts on you. It is balancing energy *in* with energy *out.* Like any other success in life, stress management begins within **you**. These are the principles of energy conservation.

Because social interactions account for 80 percent of our stress, I have chosen to include these definitions at the very beginning of the chapter. The basic principles throughout this handbook will be methods to conserve your resources, increase your input of positive energy, and methods to decrease output of wasted energy (extracted and never replaced).

Using these definitions as a prelude to healthy communications, it is also imperative that **assertiveness** is defined as any structured situation that eases the acquisition of emotionally expressive behavior. In order for communication to be healthy, it requires that we take ownership for what we need and how to express it. When we say what we mean and mean what we say, there is decreased manipulation and stress in our lives.

Please review Diagram 1:

NEEDS ➠ FEELINGS ➠ THOUGHTS ➠ BEHAVIOR

to clarify whether the dialog is emotional or rational. Refine your listening skills to fit this transition. When you are interacting based on *feelings*, attempt to "turn your head off and turn your heart on." Just allow your presence and attention to be the gifts you offer to the sender. Perhaps you can help each other in identifying the underlying, motivating feeling or need, and then together explore acceptable methods to satiate those basic stressors.

Stress Management

Stress provides the motivation to change behavior, and often the internal dissonance intensifies just before we *rationally* realize that we must change something either internal or external. Listening to and honoring our physiological messengers is really critical to our holistic health. Healthy communication begins within.

When we honestly say *yes* or *no* we have made a basic assertion. Have you ever noticed how much energy you truly save when you say *yes* or *no* versus *maybe* or *later*? Not only our children, even phone solicitations whittle away at us until we give in and say yes—when we really wanted to say no. Consider for a moment—what value does *yes* have if we never say *no*? How would the nature of our society change if the first word our children learned was *yes* instead of *no*? Somewhere very early in our life, these two simple words take on such ambivalent meanings.

So can we start here to clean up the debris attached to these basic affirmative replies? When can you safely begin to assert with an honest *no*? I suspect that most of us have become nearly desensitized to internal distress or violation of our core values. We just assume that this *dis*ease is a normal process. We begin to "turn off" our physiological cues and not honor our own inner truths. If we fail to trust our biological, instinctual communication, how can we know what is real within our external world?

We have much in common with the animal world; the best illustration of this is to watch a two-year-old child in a room full of strangers. The child, very much like a dog, will avoid those people who do not feel safe to them. They will gravitate to those who emit an aura of trust and safety. This brain stem function is a gift that we share with the animal kingdom; it is designed to promote our survival both internally and externally. Unlike the animal kingdom, we as humans rely on our neocortex to overrule the basic language of our body and brain. We learn to medicate or deeply deny this distress or internal dissonance.

Healthy communication requires that we first learn to listen to our own body as it tries to tell our arrogant neocortex when there is incongruence. Internal honesty begins when we enhance our internal congruence and really trust the intricate, valid feedback system that we possess. How and when we perceive a situation as a threat is largely based on our sense of competency or a positive self-concept. When we feel competent to solve, adapt, or intervene in life variables, there exists less of a threat to our safety as perceived in the brain stem.

An effective intervention at this time would be to ask yourself the following questions when you experience stress or defensiveness with the next person or situation:

What can I do to change this situation?
How important is this issue to me?
What "core value" is at stake?
What are my alternatives?
Who owns this issue/problem?
Are the energy/emotional costs of this interaction/conflict
*   worth the benefits?*
What is the real issue involved?
Is there really an issue involved here, or is this
*   predominantly a personality clash?*

We often take on crusades for social change especially within our birth families. These families are so emotion-ally-laden that the *wall* we carry around with us really distorts our vision—not to mention how very fatiguing it is to carry around a six-foot thick wall.

Almost every family has "crazy-makers" in it. The essence of health is not to *change* them but to change our response to them. This means that we have to honor the multitude of lessons which people and events have specifi-cally taught us.

This is not acceptable to my sanity, safety, values.
I am not comfortable with this situation.
I choose not to keep repeating this distress.

Sometimes the healthiest thing that our adult **self** can do for our emotional **self** (child within) is to detach or divorce our birth family.

When the battle for our ideal becomes harshly defeated by reality, it is often in our own best interest to set down the *wall* and invest our energy in building windows rather than more walls. That decision is yours to make. Energy is a very precious commodity. How you choose to invest yours will determine the quality of your health and your life satisfaction.

Our relationship to our birth family greatly affects how we interface with the rest of the world. Especially how we communicate and perceive the rest of the world. Much of our inner dialog, especially self-defeating messages, is a link to unfinished business related to our birth families.

Quick Fix

To maintain accountability for both your emotions and your rational dialog, begin your internal assessment by asking these questions. When the issues seem very complicated, put the questions and replies in writing so you can sort things out:

What am I really feeling?
What is the real issue?
What is the "bottom line" here?

What hurts me the most?
What makes me dread acting on this issue?
When you're really brave ask yourself, "What am I *really*
  afraid of regarding this person/situation?"

It is human to search for a reason for everything, including our gut-level reactions. I would advise you that this is an exercise in futility because the emotions underlying your response do not have a rational basis. Your reaction is largely prompted by "old feelings" or unmet needs. The long-term benefit here would be to identify the scars and honor your history. Then decide *where* you want to begin your search for health in *how* you communicate to *self.*

Please remember that your history has sensitized you to some persons or situations. If this still has a negative influence on your emotional, social, and physical health, there is no time like today to become your own advocate.

Let's take sensitive areas like trust and respect. For many of us this may be a vague idea, or we may not know it at all, or we struggle with it constantly. If *trust* is a fledgling concept for you, based on history or experiential learning, it may be time for you to build your own healthy definition. Nurture the elements essential for *trust* to become a reality. Without a viable sense of trust, communication will forever be stressful and largely ineffective, since you will be expending most of your energy maintaining an internal defensive posture.

The elements that are essential for healthy, reliable *trust* to exist are: honesty, consistency, fairness, and emotional congruency (a person's behavior matches their words). When our history has a void of healthy role modeling of trust we either avoid ever really trusting anyone, recklessly allocate trust to people, or cultivate a dependency or conditional relationship and confuse *control* with trusting.

Keep in mind that when you are expending your energy building a defensive position or reply, it is impossible for you to *listen* to what the other person is trying to tell you. Offense and defense are excellent strategies for combat and football, yet not really productive for communication—at least not healthy, effective interaction.

Strategies for Long-Term Change

Try the following strategies for long-term change:

Choose your battles wisely.
- What can I do to change this situation or person?
- What are the energy or emotional costs of this conflict or change to me?
- Are the costs worth the benefits?
- How important is this issue to me?
- What "core values" are at stake?
- What are my alternatives?
- Who owns this problem?

Stay issue-based. When you feel the situation deteriorating or the interaction goes off on a tangent, ask aloud:
- What is the real issue here?
- What is the bottom line?
- What can *we* do to modify this situation? (Encourage team effort.)

Refocus your energy to keep issue- or task-oriented.
▸ Separate facts and feelings and avoid personality attacks.
▸ When personality issues enter the dialog, state one of the following:

My personality is not the issue here.
Specifically what measurable behavior changes do you need to see?

Develop alternate courses of action. Request "timeout" and schedule a time to resume dialog. Allow both persons time to center themselves and sort out the real issues involved. When emotions distort logical dialog, you have a reaction and not a rational response.

Reaction is based on defense-building and emotional vulnerability. Allow *self* and sender the opportunity to "save face," or to maintain their level of integrity without needless humiliation. To humiliate another human being is a control strategy and not really healthy behavior. Remember that only persons who feel inadequate, inferior, or vulnerable have a need to control. When we are confident within our*selves*, we are at ease with choice and change, and individual differences add dimension versus constriction.

Put concerns and possible solutions in written form. This approach allows both parties to "save face," reduces the emotional risk, allows all individuals time and space to deal within their own level of readiness. This approach also allows each person time to separate facts and feelings. They can rewrite the issues until they state *precisely* what they mean without the additional burden of having to deal with the nonverbal plus verbal response of the other person.

This is especially important regarding highly emotional issues; i.e., letters to your family members to discuss unfinished business, or to commend each for what they have done well. When we deal with emotions regarding family members, written catharsis provides us with new insight, explores both sides of the story, promotes growth, provides two-way feedback, and allows for closure.

Make an appointment to discuss areas of conflict. Allow yourself time to regroup, temper your emotional reaction, decrease distractors, and enhance a responsible posture.

Convert all *whys* to *what*. Change *yous* to *I*. Whys and yous elicit the child within us, and a defensive reaction. Just watch or experience how it feels when someone begins a statement with "Why are you behaving like this?" or "You make me angry." Eye pupils constrict and body posture becomes more rigid. The listener will withdraw both emotionally and physically. These simple words elicit a stress response, and cause downshifting in the brain rendering resolution next to impossible.

"I" messages allow you to take ownership for the words that follow it. No one makes you angry, this is your choice. What the other person does elicit in you is disappointment, hurt, frustration, confusion, or belittlement. Anger is never a primary emotion, rather a facade for the vulnerability that the emotions elicit. To help focus, ask yourself these questions before you put your mouth into operation:
What do I need?
What do I feel?

What do I think ?

Once answered, these questions will allow you to know and feel what you really want to say. Honesty begins within you. It is impossible to expect others to honor your feelings when you do not do so yourself.

We are all alone
In these games we play
Being it night or day
Trying to accomplish
Something, somehow, someway
No matter where we go
We are still here at play
If we enjoy each moment
Night or day
And realize our work
can be our play

By Frosty Duckson

Nutrition and Stress Reduction

3 The first two chapters addressed internal and external communication, methods to enhance the quality of these interactions, and ways of reducing the toxic by-products. This chapter will explore nutrition as the sum of all the interactions between an organism and the food it consumes. I will explain how nutritional deficits may actually elicit symptoms we label "stress reactions" or residuals and explore methods to decrease the chronic destructive impact of stress.

Blood Sugar

According to Dr. Arthur Guyton, author of *Textbook of Medical Physiology*, the absence or presence of energy in the foods you consume will largely determine how your body is prepared to respond. Many of the physical and emotional symptoms that people blame on stress, e.g., headaches, fatigue, depression, irritability, hyperacidity, and lowered resistance, may actually be a response to the foods they have consumed. Also many of these symptoms are the result of specific nutrient deficiencies. The specific fuel which your body requires for energy is glucose. In the absence of glucose, the body tissues can shift to use fats and protein for energy. However, the importance of maintaining a normal and constant concentration of blood glucose is that glucose is the only nutrient that can be utilized by the brain and retina.

Perhaps the single element most affecting our brain function is our blood sugar level. Your brain uses over 70 percent of the glucose in your body, so when your blood sugar drops below 70 mg, the first indication you will have is a decrease in visual acuity. Becoming aware of your own health legacy, especially diabetes, attention deficit disorder (ADD), premenstrual syndrome (PMS), and alcoholism, might heighten your interest in closely monitoring your brain's response to low blood sugar (hypoglycemia).

Hypoglycemia is a significant cause of most of these predispositions. At the Calgary Institute in Canada, research has proven the changes. Our blood sugar normally drops at 10 a.m. and 2 p.m., so if you would like to become more familiar with how your brain and behavior, or that of your family, is affected, these are good times to use your body like a clinical laboratory and assess the following response. Fasting blood sugar is 60-90 (the lowest you'd ever want it); your brain functions best when your blood sugar stays between 70-100.

When your blood sugar (B.S.) drops below 70, your vision gets blurry, it's more difficult to focus, it may feel like the lighting in the room has changed. This is the ideal time to intervene to prevent further dropping. When your B.S. drops below 60, your short-term memory decreases. For example, you may forget what you came in the room for, where you left your keys, or what you were saying in the middle of a sentence. When your B.S. drops to 50 you become increasingly irritable and unable to assimilate new information, no matter how many times you reread it. The best illustration of this would be rush-hour traffic at 4 p.m. when most drivers have a B.S. of 40-50; this is also why happy hours are such a success—we crave alcohol or sweets when our B.S. drops below 60. Our body has a mind of its own. When the brain is deprived of its main fuel, it will be attracted to the most rapid sugar fix such as alcohol and sugar.

Premenstrual drop in estrogen greatly affects our blood sugar, so it is in our best interest to stabilize it the best we can to avoid the dramatic consequences.

It is also interesting to note that if our B.S. drops normally at 10 a.m. and 2 p.m., these are the times that many of our students tend to have their core subjects, e.g., math and science. So, if you want to honor your family's ability to learn and avoid agitated behavior, perhaps one of the best places to begin would be to consider a snack every three hours throughout the work day. There are times when we do not have access to refrigeration for perishables or temperature control is an issue. In these situations I recommend a nonperishable snack such as the one in the next Quick Fix.

Place the ingredients in a zip-lock bag, and locate the bag in your knapsack, briefcase, or desk drawer. A fringe benefit, besides optimizing your brain's ability to assimilate and effectively cope with all the stimuli, is when you stabilize your blood sugar, your body burns cleaner and leaves behind less toxic buildup, i.e., adipose, cholesterol deposits, and acidity.

It is more physiologically efficient for us to consume six small meals each day rather than two large meals. This nutritional approach reduces sluggishness from 1,000 calorie heavy meals, when your blood supply is routed to digestion and away from your brain. Small frequent meals, i.e., grazing, also reduces indiscriminate eating which increases when we are overly hungry.

Quick Fix

I recommend the following "power pack" because it includes fiber that delays the body's production and release of glucose. It has a rich source of amino acids that are critical to every hormone and enzyme that your body manufactures. Best of all it's tasty and not messy.

Use ⅓ of each of the following:

raw almonds or filberts (the harder the nut the lower the fat content), raw because the oils and roasting process destroy some of the nutrients

raisins, cranraisins, and dates as rich sources of iron and fiber

any cereal that is a good source of bran to lower cholesterol.

This combination provides 200 calories/large handful times two. It does not matter what the temperature is; this mixture will be attractive and tasty, and maintain your blood sugar.

You will find that when you stabilize your B.S., your brain will function better, you will get less hungry, avoid indiscriminate snacking (junk foods that are high in fat or salt), and decrease cravings for alcohol and sweets. Not to mention that you enhance your ability to cope and you will be less irritable. When you are less irritable you will be better able to cope, have a healthier perception, and increase your patience.

I have introduced this chapter with emphasis on the significance of blood sugar because decreased short-term memory and irritability warp how we cope with any stressor. Often these effects are confused as a response to stress when in fact there is a metabolic cause. It is easy to reverse *once you listen to your own body.* It amazes me at how readily we'll use medications to allay these symptoms rather than heeding the message our physical vehicle is attempting to tell to us.

I do believe this passive approach to our health care requires revision. Allowing our minds to listen and *pay attention to* what our bodies are trying to tell us creates the mind-body connection. In stabilizing our blood sugar we avoid visual deterioration, damage to neocortical cells (thinking brain cells), decreased demand on our pancreas, and a multitude of metabolic imbalances. When we stabilize our blood sugar, we also enhance our immune system, which is greatly compromised with the impact of stress.

Genetic Legacy

Before we proceed, I would encourage you to find out which illnesses have been the primary cause of death for the two generations of family before you. The answer will let you tailor the rest of this chapter to fortify your genetic weaknesses. You will be best able to identify your "weak organ" as your genetic legacy. As Dr. Deepak Chopra explains in his book, *Perfect Health*, this is significant because it is within this "weak organ" that you will store your stress. Applying logic here this equation would look like this:

"weak organ" + stress = organ/system failure = disease = death/disability

The major (70-80%) reaction to your stress is first noticed from your shoulders up. This is the ideal time to intervene, before it gets pushed below your shoulders or lodged in your temporomandibular joint (TMJ). The TMJ connects both sides of the skull with the jaw. When we walk around with our jaws clenched and talk through our teeth rather than yell, tell our boss where to get off, or say words which may be honest yet hurt another person or our relationship with them, we restrict joint mobility. People who keep that anger or inability to verbalize their concerns locked within their mouths often continue to grind their teeth together during their hours of sleep. Keeping the TMJ locked tightly shut will result in unnecessary pressure in the joint and muscle shortening which will restrict movement and elicit pain when the jaw is moved.

The following two chapters will specifically address cognitive and relaxation strategies to reduce the negative impact of stress. The energy of stress is a profound motivator when we are aware of the challenge to act and take this action before the stress response immobilizes us. In correlating your genetic legacy and these initial indicators of stress, you can select any of the following healthy choices and "quick fixes" to reduce the negative physiological impact of the stress response.

I will organize the nutritional interventions to stress by systems and label them accordingly. This will allow you a quick index for review and the most specific interventions for your weak organ/system. I will start at the top of your body and work down and around it. Starting at the major circuit-breaker, your brain, seems expedient since it is within this neurological network that we first perceive stress and where we can defuse it.

Neurological

Of greatest significance here is the premise that stress increases the metabolic process that requires greater amounts of vitamin B complex to facilitate carbohydrate metabolism—the most immediate source of glucose. As your body uses more vitamin B, it decreases the supply available to the nervous system to regenerate the myelin sheath. The myelin sheath is the insulating wrap that protects a nerve fiber and prevents electrical artifacts within your body and brain.

Quick Fix

Supplement your diet with a vitamin B complex (to include at least 8 components listed on the back of the bottle) 3-4 times per day. I take three in the morning to optimize my energy and protect my neurological system when my physical and emotional demands are greatest. Keep in mind that vitamin B is water soluble, so whatever excess your body does not need you will urinate away. The only manifestation that you will have of large doses is that your urine will glow-in-the-dark—almost—due to the yellow color caused by riboflavin.

If you want to vividly recall what a deficiency of vitamin B complex feels like, remember the last time that you drank more than four cups of coffee, drank more than three alcoholic beverages, or took a diuretic, since each of them increases your excretion (via urination) of the B complex. Do you recall your shaking hands, heartburn, and irritability—perhaps the lights were too loud? These are all symptoms of vitamin B deficiency, not to mention frequent headaches and fatigue.

Please find a natural food source of vitamin B supplements to avoid your body's rejection of the chemicals used in manufacturing synthetic ones. Many people complain of nausea and indigestion with synthetic vitamin supplements. For all the nutrients I will suggest from this point forward, I strongly encourage you to find supplements derived from the *foods* in which they are richly found. There are many home distributors of natural vitamins. Consult your phone book for the one nearest you.

To provide you with a visual image of how nerve endings and muscle tissue interact and where nutrients are necessary, a diagram is provided on page 67. The myoneural unit conducts an electrical impulse from a nerve to a muscle or another nerve to initiate specific action.

This unit of muscle-nerve work is the area most exhausted with chronic or intense stress. At the end of the synaptic knob there are tiny pores that allow the transmitter substance to leave the nerve, enter the cleft, and convey the message to the muscle fiber. Calcium is the only substance that serves as gatekeeper for these pores and to allows adequate transmission of nerve impulses. When blood calcium concentrations fall, the nerves become hypersensitive resulting in excess muscle contractions. In contrast, high calcium concentrations depress nerve irritability.

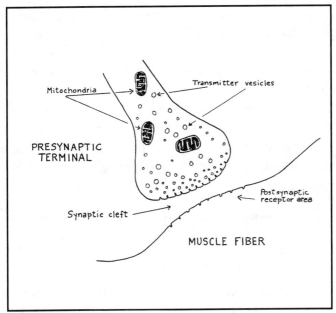

Myoneural Unit

A good illustration of serum calcium deficiency is a two-year-old child, and then at every two-year increment from then on until a child is 21 years old. During these two-year growth spurts, the long bones use all of the serum calcium for growth and bone density. Now hold this mental image of a two-year-old, how long can they sit still, and if their ears could move, every part of them would be moving.

Another example of calcium depletion is after an intense workout. The serum calcium has been used to conduct nerve-muscle impulses, and is absorbed by bone mass with weight bearing. Have you ever noticed the little spasms in your legs, arms, and face after these workouts? These little seizures are an indication of calcium deficiency, as are leg cramps, especially at night time (if your circulation is adequate). Have you ever noticed when children are in the midst of growth spurts, they also complain of leg cramps, spasms, and insomnia? These are all related to deficiency of serum calcium necessary for nerve-muscle conduction.

Dairy products are the richest sources of calcium, but also of fat and calories. Most cardiologists will advise adults to decrease their intake of dairy fats. Some adults are lactase deficient and not able to effectively metabolize dairy products.

Quick Fix

Take 200 mg of calcium, plus magnesium, phosphorus, and vitamin D. Avoid taking calcium without these other trace minerals, because it is best absorbed along with these trace minerals.

To resolve a headache, decrease tension, and promote quality sleep, take a vitamin B complex and a calcium compound (one that includes the trace minerals). Within 25 minutes watch the tension decrease. Use this combination before exercising and help your nerve-muscle units to work their best for you.

Visual Acuity

Maintaining your blood sugar between 70-100 mg will maintain visual acuity by providing this essential nutrient to the retina. If you have a family legacy of diabetes or suffer from hypoglycemia, please consider taking 15-30 mg of zinc. Zinc is the central molecule of insulin, like iron is central to hemoglobin (the oxygen carrying component of blood). When we are deficient of zinc, our pancreas is unable to produce the insulin we need.

Zinc is a trace mineral found in liver, peas, oysters, grains, beans, and nuts. Only if you eat few or none of these food sources, consider a food supplement. Zinc is joined with vitamin A to increase the supply of antibodies and is useful in curbing some allergies.

Vitamin A or beta carotene is necessary for the production and function of your visual purple. Visual purple is the purple pigment of the retinal rods which stores large quantities of vitamin A. Vitamin A is exchanged back and forth through the membranes of the rods and cones of the retina and is very important for the adjustment of light sensitivity of the receptors in the retina. A good indicator of vitamin A deficiency is acute distress in adapting with night vision. You have trouble with night vision if the oncoming lights of another auto at night causes eye pain while you attempt to adjust to the light change. Light sensitivity in general may be your own personal cue that your stores of vitamin A within the retina are depleted.

Rich sources of vitamin A are fish oils, egg yolks, and butter. Rich sources of beta carotene which is the precursor of vitamin A can be found in foods with the carotene pigment. The more intense the pigment, the higher the source of beta carotene. These yellow, orange, and red foods are carrots, pumpkins, squash, sweet potatoes, peppers, apricots, papayas, peaches, cantaloupe, and cherries.

Cardiovascular (CV)

This is perhaps the most critical system for living. It is the one most drastically and chronically affected by stress, and yet a most neglected system (at least until we've had a heart attack).

The stress response directly triggers the adrenal gland to prepare the body for "fight or flight." Epinephrine and norepinephrine are the most profoundly impacting hormones secreted by the adrenal gland. These "energizers" act on all blood vessels, causing constriction in almost all vascular beds, except skeletal and cardiac muscles where they cause dilation.

When you experience stress, have you ever noticed how your heart feels like it will jump right out of your chest? This occurs because the ventricles of your heart are pumping with as much force as they can muster. The only hazard here is that it is pumping against great resistance. Because all (except skeletal and cardiac muscle) blood vessels have constricted, the heart must pump with mighty force against smaller outlets.

Take a minute and picture a water faucet with a three -inch hose attached to it. Open the faucet wide open and feel how easily the water flows through it. Now remove the three-inch hose and attach a one-inch hose, again turn the faucet on full blast. Feel the tremendous pressure exerted against the walls of the hose—if you do not blow a hole in it!

This effect occurs within your blood vessels in the presence of adrenergic hormones like epinephrine and norepinephrine. The reason that I have presented this excerpt in physiology is to illustrate just what a pounding your CV system takes regularly and even more profoundly if your life has excessive stress in it. The following interventions will be a priority to you if you have a family legacy of CV disease. We manifest stress in our weak organ, and that would be the system failure that caused deaths in your ancestors.

Besides the relaxation strategies identified in Chapter 5, I would propose the following interventions to best fortify your CV system. Optimize the elasticity of your blood vessels by sustaining both the production and maintenance of elastin and connective tissue. Elastin and collagenous tissue are best manufactured in the presence of vitamin E plus selenium and vitamin C.

Food sources of vitamin E are safflower oil, whole grains, green leafy vegetables, wheat germ oil, egg yolk, liver, and nuts. Cooking and processing foods can substantially reduce their vitamin E content. Excellent sources of selenium are liver, kidney, meats, and seafood.

An increased level of vitamin C also decreases cholesterol in the blood and liver, increases the buildup of collagen, increases the activation of white blood cells (WBCs) and interferon, which increases your resistance to infection. Taking a vitamin E plus selenium reduces the amount of E required for a therapeutic effect because they have a synergistic effect in protecting the cell membrane and the nucleus.

Fat-soluble vitamins are vitamins A, D, and E. It is important to emphasize here that any vitamin measured in international units or I.U. is a fat-soluble vitamin, which means it is stored in your liver and fat tissues, rendering these vitamins toxic to the liver. The doses that are recommended for therapeutic intervention will not result in liver damage unless exceeded or liver damage is already present. I recommend that you **not** exceed the recommended therapeutic dose of these vitamins to avoid damage to your liver and nausea.

If you have a cholesterol level over 200, you may want to consider adding Lecithin capsules that are the richest source of choline (a vitamin B component). Choline serves as a "cholesterol detergent" by emulsifying the cholesterol and dumping it into your intestinal tract—a much safer place for it to be than collecting inside your blood vessels making them even narrower.

High density lipoprotein (HDL) also decreases cholesterol. HDL is increased with aerobic exercise or eating fish and essential fatty acids (linoleic acid, EPA, DHA).

Besides fortifying the tissues in the CV system, it is necessary to enhance its function, carrying oxygen to every cell in the human body. Deep breathing is the first step in supplying oxygen to your heart-lung exchange network at the base of your lungs. Hemoglobin is the oxygen carrying protein within your blood. It requires adequate iron supply to be formed.

Rich dietary sources of iron are raisins, molasses, spinach, and prunes. Vitamin C promotes iron absorption. I highly recommend these food sources of iron since many people have difficulty digesting an inorganic supplement (it can cause diarrhea or constipation).

Vitamin B-12, another of the vitamin B components, helps your body produce red blood cells and removes one of the causes of pernicious anemia. It is best absorbed when taken with calcium and magnesium. This combination was discussed under the neurological system—and now to think it has a positive influence on the CV system too!

I expect that you've all heard all you want to hear about lowering your fat intake! I'd like to approach this suggestion from another perspective. The stress response increases the coagulation of your blood and fatty acids decrease the viscosity leading to a strong likelihood of blood clot formation. Whenever you slow the flow of blood, you increase the formation of clots.

Decreasing your fat intake to 20 grams/day will also encourage weight loss and reduce your risk of cancer, since free radicals have a direct affinity for fat molecules. Free radicals are strongly attracted to other substances, such as polyunsaturated fats, nucleic acid in genetic codes, or cellular proteins. All these reactions increase the likelihood of abnormal cell growth leading to premature aging, cancer, decreased immune function, and atherosclerosis.

Your mental acuity also decreases with your dietary intake of fat. Your body exerts much energy and time to metabolize fat, which is why you feel sluggish the morning after you've had a high fat dinner or late night snack. Those persons subjected to severe, prolonged exposure to -40°F are perhaps the only individuals who need the insulating effects of high fat intake. Your body, like your automobile, burns cleaner (less residue on the valves and carburetor) with a diet high in complex carbohydrates and low in fat.

Please don't forget water to flush all systems of their toxic wastes especially during the hours of 4:00 a.m. to noon, which is the time your body detoxifies. This time cycle assumes that you are not a nocturnal being. If you are, then your circadian cycle will vary. But I do not think there is any misunderstanding when your body is trying to detoxify, because every excretion from your body will be very foul. Even your perspiration will be more pungent. This is an ideal time to help this process by increasing your water intake. As one becomes more dehydrated (inadequate water), the blood viscosity also decreases, resulting in the risk of easier clot formation and increased workload for the heart to pump around this sludge.

Keep in mind that one tends to loose nearly as much water from the respiratory system as through the kidneys. Perhaps you've noticed that when you are in an environmentally-controlled facility, even when you have been drinking significant amounts of water, you do not urinate as often. This is because you're losing the water out of your respiratory system as you breathe. It is ideal to urinate at least three times during this detoxifying period (from the time you awake until noon). If you do not, then reevaluate your body's ability to do the tasks it must do and, perhaps, why you feel sluggish and constipated.

Speaking of water, it is also a natural diuretic that will lower your blood pressure. Vitamin B complex is also a natural diuretic. Decreasing your sodium intake is another area I'm certain that you've heard before. As you take in more sodium, your body will hold more water, which means more volume for your heart muscle to have to pump around. Excessive volume could lead to cardiac fatigue or enlargement. Remember that as the heart gets larger there is less room for the lungs to do their work.

Explore an effective method to filter the heavy metals and bacteria out of your drinking water. Often this also improves the flavor. Coffee, tea, or alcohol do not count as fluid intake because they are diuretics, which means it will further dehydrate you. The most ideal way to enjoy your coffee is to drink 8-10 ounces of water between each cup.

Gastrointestinal System (GI)

This system is perhaps the place we "stuff" emotions and stress, also the area most deeply affected by chronic stress. Treating your GI system kindly is the first place to start. When you are under increased stress, avoid foods that irritate your stomach even under peaceful conditions, i.e., fried foods, spicy entrees, and alcohol.

Your GI system is a hollow tube running from your mouth to your anus, with a small (approximately five pound capacity) outpouching called your stomach. If all goes well, it is natural that within four to five hours after putting food into the mouth-end of this hollow tube, it comes out the anus-end as waste. The longer that waste material sits in the colon, the more impurities and toxins are reabsorbed into the blood vessels surrounding the intestinal tract. If you have ever been constipated, you are aware of how toxic you feel, and maybe even your attitude is affected. The best laxative is water; the more dehydrated waste becomes the more difficult movement along the colon is.

I caution you regarding mineral water as your source of hydration, since the minerals in the water cause water to move out of the colon by osmosis and can intensify constipation. Should you want the flavor of mineral water, as with coffee, just alternate with 8-10 ounces of water to balance this effect.

The vitamin B complex is essential to your GI system. Vitamin B1 is essential for the manufacturing of hydrochloric acid. It also increases the tone of the intestinal tract resulting in a decrease of atonic constipation. Vitamin B3 is essential for effective digestion. The balance of the B components is essential for carbohydrate metabolism, providing nutrients to the endocrine system, which interfaces directly with metabolism.

The vitamin B complex is necessary for the regeneration of the epithelial tissue (the lining of the GI tract). An indication of a vitamin B deficiency will be cracks at the corners of your mouth and lips. You may notice these symptoms especially after peak stressful times when all your vitamin B has been exhausted.

The vitamin B complex also is essential for cell reproduction, synthesis of amino acids to form body proteins and nucleic acids that combine to form DNA and RNA. It regulates body fluids by setting up a balance between sodium and potassium resulting in a diuretic effect.

If hyperacidity is a source of distress for you, please consider your calcium, magnesium, and phosphorus as a natural antacid versus ingesting an antacid that is high in aluminum (major cause of Alzheimer disease).

Some adults respond to a dairy products with hyperacidity and indigestion. If gastric distention and indigestion closely follow the ingestion of dairy products, it may be advisable to reevaluate the use of them and consider alternatives.

Immunological

As mentioned before, the adrenal gland is the focal point for the systemic stress reaction. Besides epinephrine and norepinephrine, cortisol is secreted by the cortex of the adrenal gland. If you have ever had a cortisone injection or taken cortisone, it dramatically suppresses the inflammatory reaction. When cortisol is dumped into your blood supply it suppresses the immune reaction throughout your body, largely the T-lymphocytes or the mighty warriors of the immune system. These warrior macrophages patrol your body night and day to engulf aberrant cells. Aberrant cells are chromosomal deficient, genetic errors, or cancer cells. We all have such cells in our body. However, it is the rate at which we reproduce them that determines whether healthy cells or cancer cells will prevail. Add to this dilemma the increasing presence of carcinogens in our food, water, and air supply. What is there to do?

Increase your intake of beta carotene, the precursor of vitamin A, which joins with zinc to increase the supply of antibodies. Beta carotene helps maintain normal epithelial membrane and stimulates mucous secretion, providing physiological protection against invasion of respiratory pathogens. Vitamin A is also good *health* insurance for the adrenal gland, which becomes exhausted with exposure to chronic stress. It also helps restore tissues damaged and inflamed by arthritis.

Vitamin A, E plus selenium, and vitamin C are all antioxidants, which means they decrease the formation of aberrant cells, neutralize mutagens, and decrease production of cancer cells. Vitamin E plus selenium together slow the division of cells, allowing the chromosomes to correctly divide and convey healthy genetic coding to the next generation of cells.

Decreasing your fat intake to 20 grams/day will also decrease your risks of cancer, since free radicals have a direct affinity to fat molecules. Stabilizing your blood sugar will also increase your immune response by providing the cells with the energy they need to do their jobs. It also will decrease faulty metabolism of other nutrients. Allowing your body to burn clean means fewer carcinogens produced by your own body.

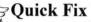

Quick Fix

Ingest the antioxidant vitamins, beta carotene, vitamin E plus selenium, and vitamin C before noon when your body is detoxifying. These antioxidants will enhance your body's ability to neutralize or eliminate cancer causing toxins. This is especially significant if you have a family legacy of cancer. Vitamin E plus selenium is essential especially if you have a family history of breast cancer. It is also effective for women with polycystic breast disease.

A recommended therapeutic vitamin regimen is on page 141. Select vitamin and mineral supplements which would best fortify your weak system. This would deter that system being further strained by stress. The weak organ theory, states that we hold our stress in our weak organ, assuring its failure. To take preventive action, making some healthy revisions in your nutritional approach, and decreasing the detrimental impact of stress are very critical choices for you to make. I will illustrate the physiological rationale and present the choices to you.

Enhancing Your Brain Power

I can imagine that many of you have heard that "fish is brain food." What are your chances if you do not like fish? Does your brain starve? Let's explore amino acids (which are the products of protein metabolism) and what effect they have on brain chemistry and behavior. Most of us would like to increase our attention span, accelerate our thought process, and improve our short-term memory.

It may be surprising to you to correlate what you thought was a nutritious breakfast, and the resultant sedation that a high carbohydrate meal induces. In essence, have your waffles, French toast, cereal, or pancakes for your evening meal instead of at the beginning of the day. These rich carbohydrate meals in addition to baked potatoes, rice (long grain or brown), pasta, and squash are effective at eliciting sleep. Sedation is rarely an honored or compensating vocational asset.

Foods high in tryptophane (amino acid) are turkey and popcorn. Tryptophane is a precursor of serotonin, which is a brain transmitter substance and is a major antidepressant. Tryptophane also induces sleep. Have you ever noticed how everyone needs to lie down and take a nap after Thanksgiving turkey dinner?

Another way to increase your serotonin production, especially to decrease depression, is to absorb at least 25 minutes of sunlight before noon.

The amino acid tyrosine increases your ability to focus and your level of alertness. Ideally, these foods are best to consume during the daytime hours when you need to have your brain function at peak performance. A protein rich breakfast might consist of low-fat yogurt, whole grain toast topped with ricotta cheese, or cottage cheese and melon.

Other moderately rich sources of tyrosine are natural peanut butter, eggs, mozzarella, almonds, lentils, beans, and peas. The richest sources of tyrosine are orange roughy, tuna, salmon, chicken breast (without the skin), sardines, and veal. These foods will force you to think. Now just recall the last time that you had any of these food items before bedtime? Do you recall lying awake planning the next week, wondering whom you could call, wanting to dialog an idea, or just ended up journaling or typing rather than attempting to put your mind to sleep?

Decreasing your fat intake is very significant since fats interfere with the brain's use of these essential proteins. Consider cheddar cheese as high in fat and replace it with mozzarella or Parmesan, which are lower in fat and healthier for your brain's functioning.

Foods high in tyramine elicit adverse effects in some individuals like an increase in blood pressure, migraine headaches, and anxiety or panic attacks. This would be very significant for any person recovering from substance abuse, since this myriad of symptoms closely parallels those of withdrawal.

Just think how many children and adults ingest anti-anxiety medications when in fact it very well may be due to the foods they are eating. It would be more conservative to evaluate your dietary regime and revise your diet versus medicating the side effect of the food. Again this is a **choice**.

Especially significant here would be those individuals who have invested much energy and emotion into recovering from substance abuse, and then find that an amino acid could make them physically recycle this process. This cluster of symptoms closely resembles those of withdrawal.

The medical model also treats migraine headaches vigorously. If any of your readers have suffered from migraines or love someone who does, then perhaps this part alone will pay for the book! The foods that are high in tyramine are the following:

▸ aged cheddar cheese
▸ pickled herring

- canned figs
- ripe bananas (once they have brown freckles turn them into compost since tyramine does not bake or freeze away; banana bread won't work)
- ripe avocados (these are the ones used to make guacamole—so sorry), the firm green ones are okay just like the green tipped yellow bananas
- eggplant
- soy sauce
- meat tenderizers
- Chianti

I would encourage you to do a dietary assessment especially for those individuals, for your hyperactive children, and for those with attention deficit disorder. It is sad to think that our bodies try desperately to tell us what toxins (including the very food that we eat) they are attempting to reject. What could possibly happen to the quality of our total health, if our logical self were to heed the messages that our physical vehicle tries to convey to us? The essence of this question is that there is a profound mind-body connection, and only when we honor this unity can we embark on our journey and search for wellness and health.

If you would like more detailed information, please read the references listed in the back of the book. Then I invite you to decide if this is worth the financial investment.

Choices

This is a new day, mine to use, to fill, to live
    as I see fit.
How it unfolds is up to me, the choice is mine.
I can be miserable or I can have a great day.
I can doubt or I can have faith.
I can feel depressed or I can express the joy
    that is inherent within me.
I can fear or I can trust...myself, others, God.
I can complain about aches and pains,
    or I can affirm God's perfect life within me.
I can dwell on loss or I can seek new interests,
    new joy in living.
I can criticize others or I can accept and bless them
    and enjoy happy and harmonious relationships.
I can harbor old grudges or I can forgive.
I can speak of lack or I can affirm
    God's never-failing supply.
I can give up or I can make a fresh start.
I can go it alone or I can depend on God.

by Judy Walz.

"Choose this day whom you will serve." Joshua 24:15

Cognition and Behavior

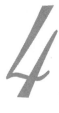 This chapter will ease your access to your "thinking brain" or your neocortex, and optimize further ascent to the uppermost lobe of your brain—the frontal lobe. The frontal lobe is where you perform long-term planning and consider future alternatives. Stress stimulates an increased level of cortisol (described on page 65), that decreased your "relaxed alertness." What this means is that as you perceive a threat and autonomically trigger the "flight or fight" stress reaction, the endocrine discharge narrows your perceptual field. This "tunnel vision" inhibits your ability to see interrelationships and you "downshift" to more primitive areas of the brain.

Optimizing Your Cognitive Capacity

If your logical capacity and cerebrate productivity happens to be the first and primary component of wellness that you wish to revise, I will provide you with information to increase your awareness of this "downshifting." I also will offer workable components for change that address cognition specifically.

The first step is to become aware of what and who you perceive as a threat. You will become internally sensitized to the feeling of putting your blinders on—or feeling a veil fall over your thinking abilities. Let's explore an example.

Have you ever noticed what happens in your thinking brain when you have someone hovering over you wondering why you have not produced more work? Or what happens when you get six different orders simultaneously? How about when someone is simply being obnoxious, unreasonable, or autocratic with their demands? It becomes harder for you to focus on the task in front of you. Your attention to details and accuracy decreases, the energy required to focus is greater, and usually you have a residual sense of being attacked or challenged.

We can be flexible and competent at multiple tasks at once when there is an environment of respect, teamwork, and loyalty. However, when the demands are indifferent, aggressive, and chronic, the result is usually one of intimidation and detachment. The impact that these invasive, unreasonable demands have on your cognitive capacity is largely based on your sense of personal worth, your self-concept, and your communication skills (both internal and external). That is the rationale for discussing interventions to fortify these components of wellness before addressing your cognitive behavior.

Quick Fix

The first step in effectively using your cognitive capacity is to separate the task from the egos involved. Both internally and of the challenger ask, "Exactly *what* do I need to do?" Remain focused on the task and avoid involving the personality of the challenger. If the challenger uses body language that makes you feel extremely subordinate, then stand up and listen to the request, or avoid eye contact with the challenger. Instead envision the person as a fax machine spitting out more information. Disengage purposefully from assault or internalization of this dump. Requesting time frames for realistic completion and prioritization of the assignments can be effective. Often it is visually centering to place a large block calendar in front of the challenger and yourself. Write the projects and due dates right onto the calendar. This strategy allows both of you (or even with a task group) to *see* what needs to be done instead of only feeling it. Clarify this overload with task-specific questions, and define which tasks can be deleted, delegated, or delayed. These "three Ds" apply to every aspect of our life and the responsibilities that confront us on a daily basis. Ask the following:

▸ *Which of these tasks or demands can be deleted?*

▸ *What can be delegated? Who can I trust to complete this well and on time?*

▸ *Which endeavors can be delayed?*

► *What do you want the product to look like?*

► *Which of these assignments do you need first?*

Most likely the answer to the last question will be "all of them," especially during this current corporate epidemic of "more for less." I believe that the incidences of injury and accidents in the workplace, not to mention the increase in substance abuse during the work day, have increased in response to this "urgency" epidemic. However, to move beyond this editorial comment, we still need to produce to maintain any level of job security. It is important to correlate the incidence of accidents to the "downshifting" that occurs with acute stress. This happens because when we are stressed our perceptual field narrows. Then we fail to see the interrelatedness of events or to foresee the consequences of our actions.

Explore what an *ideal* stress level is for you. It is at this ideal level that your mental acuity peaks and even energizes you to act more efficiently. Have you ever noticed how you procrastinate with some tasks until the deadline is on top of you? Many people express their tendency to "act better under pressure."

This cognitive game is a delicate balance, or dangerous roulette, because living on the edge can be productive for the short-term. However, the long-term effect will be adrenergic drain and disease. This rush of adrenaline in response to pressure can become your best friend or your worst enemy. Only you know what is saturation-level for you. There are many tasks that have become routine and do

not require our conscious effort. However, there are tasks
that do require our focused attention for accuracy and
safety purposes, and it is our responsibility to differentiate.

Quick Fix

Incorporate *recess* into your work day. Have you ever noticed how much energy you have with the thought of play? Take a walking lunch break, remove yourself from the work site, and savor solitude. Please avoid business luncheons where the stress escalates and defeats effective digestion process. Find a park that is near work and go there for lunch. Explore the possibility of space in the workplace for a rebounder, an exercise room. Help get membership at a fitness club proximate to work as a perk for superior performance. The exercise will increase your endorphins, ease the absorption of your excess epinephrine, and increase circulation to your brain.

Once you incorporate creativity and the opportunity to *recreate* into your work day, you will be amazed at how much better your cognitive capacity performs. Even try taking the stairs versus the elevators during the work day. This simple intervention allows you to defuse and increase your focused attention.

These actions will dissipate the anxiety, and allow you time to identify the threat to your integrity. Maybe you can even identify methods to resolve the issues. Correlate this situation to your past and feel the similarities. It is only then we identify these connections or parallels that flip the same old switches and elicit the same defensiveness and threats. The characters change. However our internal response is the same as when we were 6-10 years old. I strongly encourage you to do an autopsy on the next situation that feels threatening to you. Rewind your memory tape, recall the personality that prompted this sensation in you before. What makes the characters similar? Once you identify this correlation, it is possible to separate and change this conditioned response.

When you experience a flash of defensiveness or vulnerability and there does not seem to be a tangible rationale, look into your past. You may discover that the person who created this feeling has similar personality traits, projects anger, uses attacking communication skills, and uses the same body language as a person from your past. He or she may even look like that person. Usually authority figures who resemble the most critical parent figure in your past flip the same switches. This tendency becomes a familiar or conditioned response, and you will often be self-defensive before you even realize that you are reacting. I invite you to at least examine the possibility. Remember that it is safer for us to be angry with an employer than it is to confront a critical parent or a spouse because we fear the abandonment or loss of their acceptance. Emotionally it is easier for us to project disdain onto an employer, because the fourth commandment seems tattooed on our very essence.

Creativity

The significance of the "thinking brain" or the neocortex is that it is the center for creativity, language, complex analysis, formal and abstract thought, and processing our sensory data. The neocortex is 5/6ths of our "thinking brain." When we perceive a threat to our safety we "downshift" out of this area and into the most primitive parts of the brain. Unless we assume a posture of heightened awareness to *what* or *who* overloads our circuits there is no effective way to be proactive and detain this process. When you notice yourself becoming more territorial, defensive, possessive, or emotionally-driven, freeze frame—stop—for just one minute and realize that you have perceived a threat and that "downshifting" is occurring. This *self* defense is the central role of the limbic system that is the primary center of emotions. The limbic system maintains a balance between the brain stem and the neocortex. The limbic system combines messages from our inner and outer experiences and inhibits instinctual behavior.

You will notice that with this "downshifting" your memory also decreases. I have included a figure to illustrate this. Should you want more specific information regarding "downshifting" consult Caine's book, *Making Connections: Teaching and the Human Brain.*

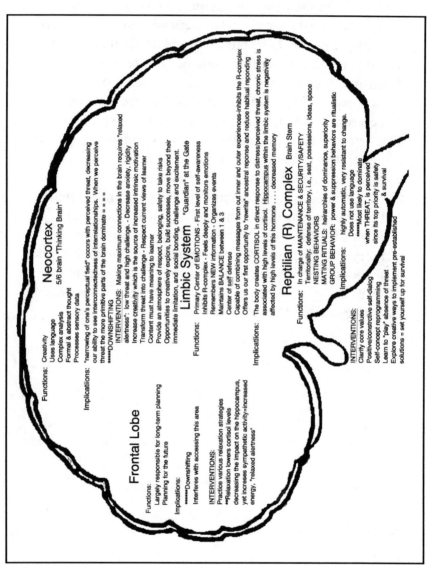

Brain Functions

In summary, to optimize access to your neocortex and maximize your cognitive abilities, it is vital to maintain a healthy sense of self and create methods to validate your positive worth. This is especially important during periods of intense stress.

Social Support

Social support is critical when external demands feel overwhelming. By social support, I in no way mean enabling co-dependency. Find those persons who know where you've been, have witnessed your successes, believe in you, and *demand* your best. These healthy support systems will not allow you to stagnate and wallow in self-pity. They will ask *what* you are going to do to modify the situation. They will help you explore your alternatives, celebrate your successes, and most of all be honest with you. Our healthy support systems serve as a mirror to reflect back to us our most positive qualities. It is this reflecting process that enables us to clarify our values, and better define our objectives. Social supports can be friends, church families, specific support groups, or recreational networking. Whatever their origination there will be some common link or mission weaving you together into the fabric of friendship.

Explore within you and your workplace avenues to incorporate creativity into your cognitive endeavors. This creative energy then becomes an intrinsic source of motivation. There are multitudes of strategies to add individuality and personal expression into the most repetitive and mundane of tasks. Examine methods to defuse potential predators, assume proactive body postures, wear clothing that makes you feel good about yourself, especially on a more stressful day.

Color

Use colors to create the energy that is most conducive to your effectiveness and to create the ambiance necessary for resolution. Remember the following:

- Purple is the color of healing,

- Blue is the color of tranquility,

- Red is the color of passion and intensity (perhaps a color to avoid if the environment is already intense), and

- Green is the color of hope.

Make note of the next time that you are talking or interacting with someone who is wearing either a purple blouse or a purple design in his tie. There is a calming effect.

Touch

The fabric that you opt to wear will also affect your internal status. It is imperative that the fabric for intense situations can breathe, i.e., natural fabrics. When you are dressing for an intense situation, avoid synthetic fabrics that make you feel suffocated even on calm days. The fabric next to your skin can also be a tangible reminder to *breathe* and to feel embraced by fluidity and complete comfort.

Summary

These are all creative alternatives to enhance your ability to feel secure, enhance creativity, and decrease anxiety. They also will generate excitement to confront a challenge as an opportunity to grow and learn more both about yourself and the environment in which you live and work. May your journey be safe, healthy, and forever growing. A journey that enables you to become everything you've ever dreamed of and even more.

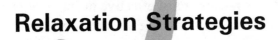

Relaxation Strategies

5   This chapter will explore methods by which you can conserve your physical self. These strategies are significant all the time, yet even more pertinent before, during, and after acute stress. I will first address the "consistently conserving" alternatives. Then I will explore with you those strategies most effective in anticipation and those for the actual throws of the stressors. Finally we will look at how to optimize your recovery to equilibrium in the aftermath. These four areas will be the manageable components, which I promised from the onset of this little book. Please feel free to begin at the area that has greatest priority for your health, and one that will give you choices for a more effective resolution.

Consistently Conserving Strategies

Awaking each morning and getting out of bed is a consistent variable. Yet this act alone is a drastic physical trauma. During sleep your metabolic process decreased up to 20 percent, your blood pressure decreased to 80/50 (very relaxed skeletal muscles lead to decreased resistance of blood flow), and your heart rate was around 50 (due to a decrease in sympathetic/epinephrine effect). For a moment envision this flaccid, near dead body, lying flat, and breathing very slowly while asleep.

Now image the startle-shock response when the alarm goes off! The few hours before your usual time to awake your brain is engaged in dream work. So when the alarm goes off, it feels like an intruder broke and entered your space. The physical response is equal to the actual response of an attempted "break and enter." The adrenergic rush raises your blood pressure, drastically increases your heart rate, and unfortunately your respiratory rate is still very slow. Therefore, the oxygen saturation of this surging blood is low. This creates a near panic attack due to lack of oxygen to your brain. It also creates heart palpitations due to insufficient respirations and oxygen delivery.

As if this was not drastic enough, then you attempt to bolt out of bed! This act alone moves 114 muscles that have been deeply flaccid. This daily, or at least five days out of the week, ritual leaves you light-headed, nauseous, and your heart ready for a real emergency. If you would really like to have a healthy body last you for 80+ years, I suggest that you learn from your cat or dog how to naturally adapt your body for this morning trauma.

Quick Fix

Take five minutes to do the following exercise before darting out of bed. Take a deep breath and stretch one leg; as you stretch this leg slowly exhale. Then take another deep breath and stretch the opposite leg. Take a third breath, stretch your arm, and slowly exhale. With your fourth deep breath, stretch the opposite arm and slowly exhale.

Change from lying to sitting at the edge of the bed. Then take a deep breath and stand upright. Five deep breaths (taking twice as long to exhale as inhale) will match a resting heart rate of 72, which is your ideal heart rate for this ritual. These five deep breaths load each of your red blood cells with as much oxygen as they can possibly carry. Please take the time to notice how your body responds to this conserving strategy.

This Quick Fix stimulates the baroreceptors (nerve receptors in the walls of great arteries of the upper body, especially the bifurcation region of the carotids and the arch of the aorta). These receptors enhance your body's ability to adjust to the blood reallocation to your brain and your heart muscle, which is essential to move 114 muscles and decrease the orthostatic hypotension. Orthostatic hypotension happens when your blood pressure drops significantly as you stand upright resulting in severe light-headedness, dizziness, and even nausea. These hemodynamics are very important to the long-term health of your heart and your brain.

Fortification for Stress

The following breathing exercise is effective in every aspect of living and managing stress without eliciting the hypoxic response. Hypoxia means not enough oxygen is available to tissues in your body. The brain is one of the first affected due to its rapid metabolism and demands for oxygen as a vital nutrient. The first sign of oxygen defi- ciency to your brain is anxiety. As the deficit intensifies it escalates to panic. It is amazing how readily both physi- cians and consumers will use anti-anxiety medications to allay the anxiety rather than treating a major cause of anxiety—lack of oxygen. This exercise will curtail an asthmatic attack and even eliminate the need for epineph- rine. I have utilized this technique with people in the emergency room and had them ask "Why hasn't someone taught me this before? This is so simple and it makes sense."

Before I explain the technique, let me review just a little anatomy and physiology regarding your heart and lungs. There are essentially three lobes or sections within your lungs. The upper lobe is above nipple line, the middle lobe is at nipple line, and the lower lobe (and perhaps the most critical space) is below nipple line and just above the lower edge of your ribs. Within this lower lobe the bronchioles resemble broccoli in structure, with alveolar sacs at the end that are airway pockets. These alveolar sacs are richly surrounded by capillaries, which is where oxygen and carbon dioxide exchange places. The walls of these sacs are elastic and balloon-like, and the longer the sac remains full of fresh oxygen the more is absorbed into the capillaries. The oxygen then goes through your heart to your brain and every other tissue that has a blood supply. The illustration below will show you this critical capillary-alveolar unit.

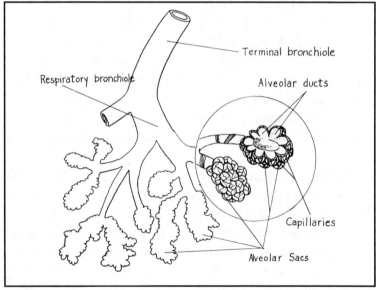

Capillary-Alveolar Unit

Your respiratory rate and depth are the first physical cues of stress. Notice your breathing the next time that you are experiencing stress, if you are breathing at all! Many people, when confronted with acute stress, fail to breathe. If they do, their breaths are very rapid and shallow. Then scant to none of the new oxygen supply reaches the alveolar sacs.   Recall the last acute stressor, perhaps when a child darted out in front of your car. You responded rapidly, left rubber on the street, and maybe your teeth were stuck in the dashboard. Yet the child was safe. Now do you remember how your brain, heart, stomach, and thigh muscles felt? Was your head throbbing, your heart about ready to jump out of your chest, stomach queasy, and every muscle aching? Largely what you were experiencing was lactic acidosis, a result of anaerobic (without oxygen) metabolism. There are people who experience this myriad of symptoms daily due to chronic stress and have antacids and aspirin as standard fixtures in their briefcase or desk drawer. Learning to breathe properly would be less expensive, consistently conserving, and enable your brain to operate more effectively. I invite you to try this. It's a wonderful strategy to teach your children before taking an exam, giving a presentation. It's best use is before attempting problem-solving or conflict resolution—maybe even any meaningful dialog.

Quick Fix

As you are learning this technique and experiencing each lobe of your lungs filling to capacity, sit in an upright position or lie flat allowing yourself maximum lung capacity, muscle relaxation, and focused attention. Close your eyes and exhale to empty your lungs. Through your mouth and nose inhale to the count of one to fill the top lobe. Then inhale to the count of two to fill the middle lobe. At the count of three inhale so deeply that it feels like you've sucked in the furniture. This process of one-two-three should be one long continuous inspiration and resemble pulling the tide in while feeling each lobe filling.

Once your lungs are fully inflated, purse your lips as if you were blowing out birthday candles and exhale. Exhale very slowly and from the top down as if your lungs were an accordion. Slowly exhale to the count of six, taking twice as long to exhale as you did to inhale. This approach allows the alveolar sac to remain inflated as long as possible, enhancing the transfer of oxygen into the capillaries. This is called 1:2 breathing (the count of three as you inhale and the count of six as you exhale).

As you acquire ease and spontaneity with this process, you can do it anywhere and anytime when you notice anxiety. Taking 3-5 breaths using the 1:2 sequencing will fully oxygenate your brain, heart, and body. You will experience relaxation of your skull muscles, decreased facial tension, and the speed of your dialog will diminish.

The tranquility that you will experience with three such breaths will equal the physical effect of a tranquilizer. I sincerely hope that the breathing exercise is even more addictive and it will cause positive physical changes. I have addressed the breathing exercise as the very first relaxation technique. Without oxygen to body tissues, relaxation is not possible.

Try this breathing exercise at bedtime and notice how the quality of your sleep improves. Practice while driving and notice how your patience and response time is affected. Always use 1:2 breathing before any important interaction to enhance the effectiveness of your brain in making connections.

As a long-term investment in your*self*, couple positive, or at least constructive, affirmations to your inhalations and exhalations. Breathe in hope and new energy, exhale doubt and fear. Breathe in life and focus, exhale ownership and hurt. The very word for lungs, pneumo, comes from the Greek word pneuma which means soul, spirit. Remember the last time you observed a child using breath-holding as an attempt to avoid feeling. Breath is our connection to our spiritual self and to breathe effectively is to honor the body's cues that something may need to be altered or avoided. To couple affirmations to the breathing enriches this awareness and the "letting go."

Quick Fix

Identify which music soothes you and creates a sense of tranquility. Music that has a waltz tempo (1-2-3) correlates to your heart sounds, brain waves, and peristalsis, which moves food through the digestive tract.

Also try pursuing music therapy which facilitates right-left brain (or cross brain) balance. There are a multitude of artists who have achieved this objective; examples are Kitaro, Danny Wright, David Lanz, Enya, Narata Samplers, George Winston, Environments, Clannad, Andreas Vollenweider, and Yanni. Listen to a musical instrument which evokes a desired emotional status within you. For example, if a harp, piano, saxophone, or guitar elicits joy or serenity, then choose the instrument and become aware of the emotion which evolves in association with each.

Sound therapy is an effective method of resting your brain, balancing interbrain neural activity, or creating the emotional state that you want. Sound pollution is a very subtle source of dissonance; for example, notice the rate and volume that everyone at your dining table consumes based on the nature of the music in the background.

The old expression of "music has charms to soothe a savage beast" is close to reality. Increasing your awareness of which sounds create stress within you and seeking out music that yields a sense of tranquility or aliveness can promote sensory balance and decrease your internal biorhythmic dissonance—stress. Sound and music can create the internal environs most conducive to supporting and nurturing your tranquility, increase focusing, or even energize you—even to be your "jump-start" in the morning.

I invite you to become increasingly aware of the internal impact of each musical instrument as you listen to it. Identify which emotion the piano leaves within you. What does the guitar or saxophone elicit? The flute usually liberates our inner child and we feel the need to whirl about, to be the most beautiful ballerina. O.K., O.K., so I have delusions of grandeur. Certain compositions allow you to feel levitation and fluidity, and aren't these the very essence of ballet and optimum creative energy? When you need such enthusiasm and playful creativity, explore which music encourages these powerful motivators for you. Many people find that gospel music is deeply inspirational, and that it allows them to feel very connected to their Higher Power. Become aware of the sounds in your work place, home place, and when you seek solitude. Define for yourself which of those sounds creates positive emotions, and those which make you feel tense or agitated.

Laughter is a marvelous stress reducer. It is impossible to laugh and have tense skeletal muscles. Laughter is like internal jogging that leads to increased digestion, increased secretion of catecholamines (alertness hormones), increased heart rate and circulation, increased respiratory activity and blood oxygen saturation. Have you ever noticed in situations where stress accumulates or peaks, how very much you appreciate that person whose sense of humor breaks the tension? Perhaps that is why the TV series *M.A.S.H.* is such a success. When the atrocity of the situation could otherwise render the surgical team impotent, their warped humor and capers inject laughter instead of hysteria and tears.

There are situations in which humor is a necessity for survival emotionally, and then seasons of the year in which humor is essential.

Quick Fix

Prepare a humor packet for someone you love—maybe even yourself. Purchase a video that is hilariously "knee-slapping," a sound track that generates laughter, or a book of your favorite cartoons. I strongly recommend videos of your favorite cartoon characters. Remember how the Roadrunner, Sylvester the Cat, Bugs Bunny, and Tweety create laughter and childlike renewal?

Visual imagery can be very effective for adjusting your mind frame, shifting your orientation to a serene location, and promote micromanagement of your energy resources. As you recall the most beautiful, mesmerizing retreat or vacation spot, what memory comes vividly to mind? Try to focus only on the natural beauty. Avoid imagery that includes people, because the emotional attachment to the memory can be contingent on the social connection versus your internal connection to the seascape/landscape.

Where did you first experience your most profound visual orgasm? (Please define orgasm as a peak sensory experience.)

Where were you when the vision before you filled your heart with such joy that you thought you'd burst?

What were the colors dancing in front of you?

Recall the last sunset or sunrise that was "sensory overload." Identify all the colors you remember—the purple, crimson, multiple shades of orange. The radiance was almost tangible.

Remember the last time you watched the sunlight create prisms through the clouds, cascading brilliant illumination?

What were the colors in the sky? Colors of plants and trees?

Which visual memories of great tranquility involve water? Waves?

I strongly encourage you to develop a "visual card file" to create mini-vacations, and elicit vivid, positive, and rejuvenating memories. Record a visual memory which makes you feel cool and refreshed.

Select one which warms you inside and outside.

Describe the most serene, inspirational place you've ever been.

Select a visual memory that validated your lovability.

What and where is the location in which you feel most spiritual?

Which sounds embraced and cradled you?

Were birds singing? Wind blowing? The sound and smell of rain? Snowflakes? Clouds?

Which fragrances still evoke belonging and security? (For me, it will always be the fragrance of yeast breads baking because Granny loved to bake bread.) Usually warm fragrances linger longer in our memory bank; e.g., the smell of drying clothes in the sun, furrowing earth, ironing clothes, or baking cookies. These memories will still elicit positive memories of family and friends. I encourage you to journal those fragrances which conjure pain or sadness and set them aside for therapeutic intervention. Much post traumatic stress reaction is triggered by our sense of smell. (I've enclosed this alert as an essential professional warning.)

Now include your skin into the memory. Where could you feel the sun? Using your skin as the weather vane, what direction was the wind from?

Who is the person in your childhood who loved you in the most healthy, unconditional way? Whose touch and hugs made the whole world brighter?

I recommend that you collect a diverse set of visual images that allow you to center, smile, and recapture the joy as if it were yesterday. These visual images may be incorporated into the following relaxation strategies.

The coupling of visual imagery and relaxation will encourage your mind to trust the memory, focus your energy, and give permission to your subconscious world to enter. It is this integration and harmony which will allow you to deeply relax and not fear the suggestions because you personally have created the metaphors for focus. Try the following:

▸ Define which visual imagery optimizes your ability to cope with pending stressors.

▸ Which imagery rejuvenates you best in the aftermath of stressors?

▸ Which visual memory carries with it a bolus of spiritual energy? Find one that levitates you beyond the every-day demands, and realities.

▸ Create visual imagery which allows you to feel cool even when you are in the midst of 120 degree weather. It will enable you to feel cooler than everyone around you. When they are all perspiring, you will remain cool while savoring the visual memory/focus of a winter wonderland, huge snowflakes, and icicles.

Stress Relievers

During stressful times remember the breathing exercise. Inhale deeply and ever-so-slowly exhale. Focus in on your positive capabilities and affirmations. Practice thought stopping whenever a self-defeating dialog begins. Identify what is the *task* or *issue* that needs to be resolved.

What is the measurable behavior change needed either within you or in the other? Assign ownership. Avoid personality attacks and stay on track while resolving the challenge.

We manifest most of our muscular stress from our shoulders up. So the following exercise is most effective in oxygenating your upper cervical vertebra and extending the muscles of your shoulders and neck that tighten with stress.

Quick Fix

Sit erect with your feet flat on the floor, arms relaxed, and hands on your lap. Close your eyes, pretend that your nose is a pencil, slowly trace a large figure-8 in the air in front of you; envision your nose as the pencil drawing this 8.

Now invert the figure 8, draw it backwards, slowly—don't jerk your neck, make the movement fluid. Stop the drawing at the center.

Make the 8 smaller, and then stop. Slowly lie the figure-8 on its side, start with the larger version, and then make it smaller.

Performing this exercise will decrease eye fatigue, visual distortion, and neck and shoulder tension. This is effective if you sit in front of a computer screen for long periods, or are a student and must do much reading in a short time.

Any activity that forces your eyes and face to remain in the same position for more than 2-3 hours will result in fatigue. This fatigue is due to the immobility of C1 and C2 (atlas and axis) which are the vertebra at the base of your skull. This exercise increases not only the mobility of this area but also the circulation and oxygen delivery to everything above it.

Progressive relaxation is most effective after stress to reverse the rigidity of your muscles. The skeletal muscles are greatly affected especially as mechanism to flee the situation. Remember the stress response is one of "flight or fight" and your body prepares to do either task by activating the skeletal muscles. This hyperarousal, or mobilization of your major "mover muscles," is critical to survival when confronted by a flesh-eating predator. However, when the threat is either perceived or unavoidable, the residual of this stress response is deep muscle fatigue, muscle pain, or actual muscle spasms.

The strategy I recommend is one defined by Edmond Jacobsen, (see Samuels', *Seeing with the Mind's Eye, p. 106)* who explained that most individuals do not even recognize that a muscle is tense until they experience the contrast. A good example is to extend your fist and arm in front of you, clench the fist even tighter, make the arm muscle really tight Now let it go flaccid and relax against your side. Most of us walk around with our muscles as tight as a G-string. We become far too accustomed to this state as the norm versus a deviation from the norm.

I invite you to try the following exercise. If any area of your body is painful, please use this information to decide where you hold the greatest amount of chronic muscle tension. Unless there is an underlying skeletal problem the muscle is irritated from the state of sustained tightness and reduced circulation. When skeletal muscles are tense, they act like a tourniquet and diminish, if not curtail, blood flow past the tense tissues.

Quick Fix

Progressive Relaxation

o   Sit or lie flat on your back without a pillow under your neck.

o   Take your deep 1-2-3 breaths.

o   Point your toes out and down.

o   Arch your foot.

o   Tighten your calf muscles.

o   Tighten your thigh muscles.

o   Suck your navel in to touch your back (oh, well, then as far in as you can pull it in).

o   Tighten your buttocks so tight you lift yourself off the surface.

o   Hold all these muscles really tight.

o   Now relax them all.

o   Clench your fists.

o   Tighten both lower arm muscles.

o   Look straight ahead and slowly lift your shoulders up toward your ears.

o   Clench your teeth.

o   Press your tongue against the roof of your mouth.

o   Scrunch up your facial muscles as if it were a wicked, monster-face.

o   Hold all these muscles taunt.

o   Slowly relax each muscle and go limp. You should feel a tingling sensation within your fingers as blood rushes to them.

Identify where you feel the greatest warmth. Which muscles hurt when you tightened them? Does this exercise allow you to feel the difference between a tense muscle and a relaxed one?

This is a good exercise for people with chronically cold hands and feet; often tension is the source of compromised circulation in them. (Being chronically cold can also be due to low blood sugar, anemia, or circulatory disease.) People with TMJ or temporomandibular joint pain may want to try this exercise to relax their muscles. Often people with TMJ spend much of their waking and sleeping hours with their teeth clenched, desperately wanting to tell someone "where to get off" or "where to stuff it." Progressive relaxation might be very beneficial to them. It may even save having ten years ground off their teeth by the dentist or, worse yet, have surgery to correct a problem that may be stress related. This exercise is a conservative alternative, it is reversible, and it will not cost anything other than time and focused intent.

We are all living in an era of great uncertainty, many changes, and much pressure to do more with less. Stress and challenge are an ever present reality. I have proposed these strategies as a gift that you can give yourself and those you value in an attempt to conserve your human resource.

Quick Fix

Spontaneous Relaxation Techniques

o Contact a friend who likes to laugh and play.
o Wear clothes that make you feel good.
o Take a walk, talk to the trees, and whistle to the birds.
o Sleep enough for *you,* take naps when you can.
o Don't take yourself too seriously. Blessed are they who laugh at themselves for they will never cease to be amused.
o Take a candlelight bubble bath with a glass of wine.
o Do something that you have always wanted to do.
o Guilt is taught—let it go.
o Don't confide in people you don't trust.
o Anticipate stressful situations and prepare for them.
o Recognize your limitations.
o Laugh and learn.

6

Sexuality, Boundaries, and Spirituality

6 At first glance these words appear very separate and exclusive of each other. They represent biological definition, social parameters, and spiritual connectedness. Each is a dimension of our sense of personal worth, safety, and ability to love and be loved. The ease with which we pursue living and truly loving uses these very ideas as the hub for momentum. When our actions have continuity, relevance, healthy relatedness, and synergism, we move through life with ease and grace. Each serves as a vital link to the other. Often it is difficult to tell one from the other. Yet it is critical to understand the basis, evolution, and nurturing of each of these concepts to obtain, sustain, and maintain health.

To integrate these social, biological, emotional, and spiritual components into one's self-concept is more a challenge of unlearning than learning. We are born as sexual beings and we learn sexuality as a process. This process takes form in early childhood, reflecting the values of our earliest role models and the degree of constructive validation for our individuality.

I have selected this area of self-exploration and intervention because of my own clinical and personal experience. These are the areas of greatest human vulnerability, and to explore them requires established rapport, a foundation of trust and safety, and a repertoire of self-sustaining skills. Until we had explored some of these alternatives, it was not appropriate to request the level of introspection and honesty that these components require. Perhaps this chapter would not be so intense if every parent came with a pedigree in genetic excellence, or a degree in parenting and life wisdom. In reality, all parents do the best they can with the history, life experience, and communication skills they've gotten largely by trial and error.

Redesigning Script and Behavior Tapes

The primary goal of this chapter is to have you redesign your script and tapes for behavior—to most ideally define who you want to become from today forward. The majority of humanity spends far too much time blaming their past for what they've become and fearing the future and rejection. They use scant time living today to the fullest. So, if you're ready, I suggest the following exercises:

 Journal

Using free word association, list the single word adjectives, nouns, and verbs that enter your mind when you entertain the words below. **Caution**— avoid analyzing what they mean and just invite them to flow onto the paper. Begin with the most comfortable word for you and come back to the others as you are ready.

o Define family
o When I think of "woman", I think/feel…
o Friends are…

o A father is...
o A mother is...
o The word trust elicits...
o Religion has provided me with...
o When I think of "man", I think/feel...

I have scattered the terms for free-word association to avoid a mind set, pace your catharsis, and to prevent a compara- tive association. We all need space to center and regroup before we plunge into this oceanic, emotional reservoir. Please set this inventory aside for a few days or flip the page and read on. Just avoid a right or wrong analysis of these lists of words and emotions.

Sexuality

Our sexual personhood is a very personal identity. It is our gender identification. It is separate from behavior and events external to us. Much of our sexual identity develops as we mimic the behavior and attitude of our same gender parent, for example, how to dress; how to express our needs, feelings, and thoughts; and how to express love.

This includes both effective and ineffective behavior. If we see women as the recipients of violence and that is the norm, we mimic this role as integral to the sexual identity for men and women.

As we approach the age of ten, we more closely observe the parent of the opposite gender as a mirror to validate appropriate sexual identity for us. Even as adults we women feel more feminine when in the company of men. This is a direct result of contrast and comparison. Men as adults are more attentive to their manners and language when in the company of females, primarily because they relate differently to women than men. This broad generalization is especially true when we have a healthy sense of our sexuality, confidence within ourselves, and have not made a habit of projecting anger onto the opposite gender.

I sincerely wish that I could recommend a quick fix for this component of our identity, however, I do not believe there is a healthy one. I'm certain that many of us have used sexual conquest as a temporary "rush" and as a source of validation. Yet often the aftermath leaves us more "hollow" than before. I am convinced that the legitimacy of our sexual identity is a very introspective, highly personal, and often painful search.

This dimension of personhood is convoluted with early childhood experiences, familial role models, social values, adolescent acceptance, and religious structure/mirroring. The interaction of these variables leaves much residue even under the healthiest of circumstances. It is beyond the scope of this book to begin to address the impact of incest or sexual violence on sexual identity.

Many exercises in this chapter will help one identify personal strengths and weaknesses in sexual identity. With that information, I encourage you to consolidate your positive experiences and construct the strengths as corner stones before you consider the weaknesses. Please remember that this area of your health is critical to your happiness, and yet perhaps one of the most painful and vulnerable areas of self-improvement. So, please be gentle with yourself as you integrate the past along with today—and most significantly as you shape the destiny of your tomorrow.

Answer the following questions that are most comfortable to you first. Come back to those questions which feel uneasy later when you have gathered the positive energy and courage to *feel* the answers and travel that path.

1. At what age do you first remember sensing or knowing that there was a difference between males and females?

2. What behavior became specific to males?

3. What behavior was specific to females?

4. At what age did the rules and expectations in your family and in your social life become different for females and males?

5. How was your sexuality nurtured in childhood?

6. How did you feel about being a female or a male?

7. Who were your strongest role models for maleness?

8. Who were your role models for femaleness?

9. What are the characteristics to this day that you associate with being a lady or a gentleman?

10. How were these definitions affected by your childhood?

11. What impact did your family have on your gender identity?

12. How did your mother influence this sense of sexuality?

13. What influence did your father have on your sense of sexuality?

14. Who was your most positive male role model?

15. Who was your most cherished female role model?

16. How did the following affect your sense of sexuality?

    a.   School:

    b.   Teachers:

    c.   Playmates/Peers:

17. How did religion make you feel about your sexuality?

18. What was your source of sexual education?

19. Who in your childhood possessed the healthiest sense of his or her sexuality (as best you can remember)?

20. If you are a woman, what was your first experience with the onset of menstruation?

21. How did the people you loved most relate to you once you made the transition into puberty?

22. What expectations changed?

23. How comfortable were your parents with their own sexuality?

Once you have completed the majority (80% or more) of these questions, put this catharsis aside for a few days. When you come back to it, shift from the emotional frame of reference into the logical—as if you were scanning a book for key points or preparing for an exam in school. Highlight the words or persons that recur or just jump out at you while you're in this logical mind set. Then identify the following common themes:

1. The recurring emotional words are:

2. I feel joy when I remember these people:

3. The healthiest role model for sexuality that I ever had was:

4. My history has provided me with _____ regarding my sexual identity.

5. I recognize the following voids:

6. What would I need to pursue now to establish a healthy sense of sexuality?

7. What source of validation would I accept as honest?

8. Religion has had the following influence on my sense of sexuality:

9. Where do I feel that I would like to begin?

10. My sense of sexuality has the following:

a.   Strengths:

b.   Weaknesses:

Interventions for sexual identity are a highly personal-ized agenda. The approaches are unique, as are fingerprints. Only you can decide how your sexuality influences the quality of your life and the choices that you make. If you decide that the voids or negative messages are detrimental to your long-term health, I encourage you to seek out a qualified therapist to assist you in finding your alternatives.

Establishing Boundaries

The health of our sexual identity greatly guides us in establishing boundaries that honor our personhood. When you establish your own comfort and respect for self, it is easier to trust your intuition as a direct messenger of the soul. As we learn to embrace our sense of sexual identity, we set limits and define behavior that is erosive, invasive, and injurious to that essence of our personhood.

Boundaries are the spaces between persons that define where you end and where I begin. Boundaries provide protection. They are the containers within which our identity develops. The only expert to consult in defining your boundaries is *you*, since the comfort or discomfort you experience with people and events entering your space is a somatic experience. Our insides actually churn, ache, or are spastic when certain people enter our space. Also, our respiratory and heart rate change. These all represent somatic experience.

The original boundaries are largely a result of how our primary care givers honored our space, nurtured trust, and adjusted to the child's timing instead of imposing their needs or unexpressed emotions. Boundaries begin to form from 3-6 months, and children test the balance of fusion and isolation near the age of two years old. During this time it is the primary care giver who touches the child and models respect and limits. It is this very behavior that helps the child to find out what is healthy for both their emotional and physical identity.

These parameters of safety and integrity are the very essence of boundaries. These parameters help the child to enclose *self* and resolve what is a comfortable and healthy limit. They help identify what issues and feelings belong to them versus their primary care giver. These differentiations are the basis of boundaries and greatly affect how we interact with others throughout our lifetime. Without healthy limits and enclosures we ooze into others' space and lose our*selves* in the process. Or we can grow old thinking that we only have worth when we are deeply enmeshed in another's space.

This dilemma of being without personal boundaries is often a cornerstone for co-dependency or addiction. The adult individual is still unable to separate which emotions, needs, and fears are theirs and which belong to others either currently or in their role models from early childhood. Learning how to construct a healthy "container" in which to enclose *self* is an ongoing process for all of us. For some individuals this process may require razing a faulty founda-tion and identifying healthy elements on which to construct a new foundation. It is my suggestion to do some free-word association with the following key elements as a new foundation in establishing healthy boundaries. In free word association you use whatever spontaneous and uncensored words come to mind.

1. Who has **ownership** for these feelings/needs?

2. How can I best maintain my personal **integrity**?

3. What do I **honestly** feel about this?

4. How can I be more **consistent** and **constructive** in setting limits?

5. What would be **fair** to me and to others involved?

6. Who has **responsibility** for changing this situation or to improve the dynamics of this relationship?

7. What do I need to **trust** someone?

The concepts in bold print are durable building blocks on which to construct viable boundaries. As a cathartic process, once the foundation is constructed and you are ready and willing, examine the needs, feelings, and unresolved issues from your past and list them . After these emotive contents and memories are in written form, close the jounrnal and allow some time to center. Wait a few days, do this with a supportive friend, or when it is complicated contract with a qualified therapist. With this list in hand rank which issues still consume your emotional energy or make you sad. Whichever issue is still the most draining, may need to be the first place to intervene. Then separate this challenge using the same questions and assessment tools discussed earlier.

Quick Fix

Use boundary affirmations like the following:
I can explore my feelings about any situation, person, place, or thing.

I recognize that my interpretation of my emotional response is more from my history than what is occurring.

I will not assume ownership for this negativism or fear.

I can let go of this rejection and pain.

I am responding normally to an abnormal situation.

I can say "no" to requests and expectations that diminish my integrity.

The long-term establishment and healing of boundaries require consistent self-nurturance. This includes choosing new friends who are supportive of your growth and honor your boundaries. This healing begins with setting limits with family members, defining what is *safe* for your inner self, and assessing body language (which comprises the emotive violation, an infringement of one's emotional expression, perhaps more significantly than intonation or which words are spoken). Identify which body postures elicit intimidation and make a change. A vivid example is avoiding having anyone stand over you and speak down to you. Either request that they take a seat or stand up yourself to physically establish parity and reduce the subordinancy. When a specific person or personality flip your "defensive switch," takes some time out and ask yourself:

▸ *Who does this person resemble?*

▸ *Where have I encountered this personality type before?*

▸ *What emotion does this person generate in me?*

▸ *Do I feel defensive? And if I do, what am I defending?*

▸ *How is this person violating my integrity or core values?*

Remember that boundaries enable us to defend these core values. Listing your core values again for this exercise may be insightful.

 Journal

My core values at this time are:

All of the defense mechanisms known to social sciences
and many that we invent as individuals allow us to suppress
needs and feelings until we have the energy to resolve or
confront them. We use denial for short-term relief. We
often repress emotional and spiritual pain until it sneaks
into our lives through dreams or manifests itself in physical
symptoms. There is an epidemic of projection during this
era of intense competition and economic insecurity.
Projection is another person dumping their manure into
your space to avoid taking ownership for their deficiencies.
The key to long-term change regarding projection is to
identify those characteristics of a manure-spreader.

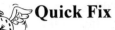 **Quick Fix**

Identification and Deactivation
of a Manure-Spreader

Toxic spreaders have the following traits:

noncommittal, wishy-washy personalities
infrequent eye contact
indirect directions or requests
fidgety body language
excessive sweetness before the "dump,"
use "suck-up" tactics to elicit subjects for potential
    dumping sites
say one thing and do another
inconsistency
unhappiness

Once you can identify the manure-spreader early in its
approach you can make the choice to reject its load with
any of the following affirmations:

I can't receive this toxic waste; my landfill is full.
I'm not authorized to handle toxic waste.
I've already fertilized my fields, thank you though.

    These playful affirmations can be said internally or out
loud depending on how comfortable you are with the
spreader. I have proposed these affirmations to workplace
teams. They have used them with each other and had fun
identifying spreaders together, and then coming up with

their own creative, curtailing, or limit setting "I" statements. "I" statements reinforce your own awareness,
celebrate your proactive approach, and acknowledge your
boundary healing and limit-setting behavior.

Defense mechanisms operate unconsciously, and are
employed by the individual to feel relief from emotional
conflict and freedom from anxiety and responsibility. When
these mechanisms are chronically, consciously, and consistently used, they truly become the essence of "crazy
-making" behavior.

Allow yourself and others to use these defenses when in
a crisis or a very painful transition as a natural coping
mechanism. It is, however, important to be aware of the
duration of their use. It can become destructive rather than
constructive adaptation. A brief rule of thumb regarding
loss, change, and adaptation, is to allow up to six months of
healing and internal processing. Of course the nature and
significance of the loss will intensify this six-month period.
The lesser the loss or more resilient the person, the less
time this healing process will require.

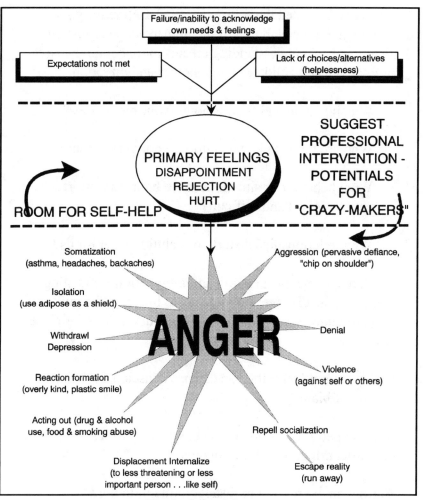

Failure/inability to acknowledge
own needs & feelings

Expectations not met

Lack of choices/alternatives
(helplessness)

PRIMARY FEELINGS
DISAPPOINTMENT
REJECTION
HURT

SUGGEST
PROFESSIONAL
INTERVENTION -
POTENTIALS
FOR
"CRAZY-MAKERS"

ROOM FOR SELF-HELP

Somatization
(asthma, headaches, backaches)

Aggression (pervasive defiance,
"chip on shoulder")

Isolation
(use adipose as a shield)

Withdrawl
Depression

ANGER

Denial

Reaction formation
(overly kind, plastic smile)

Violence
(against self or others)

Acting out (drug & alcohol
use, food & smoking abuse)

Repell socialization

Displacement Internalize
(to less threatening or less
important person . . .like self)

Escape reality
(run away)

Evolution of Anger

I have included the following as a baseline for your growth and understanding of the human adaptive response. Ideally, a basic understanding creates more comprehensive alternatives and validates your choices and direction.

Which people and friends honor your boundaries?

Who are the people who nurture your very essence?

What behavior or situations make boundary efforts compromised and difficult?

What relationships distort your ability to set limits?

Perhaps one most significant intervention for healing boundaries is discovering methods to interrupt the guilt-shame-blame cycle. Some of my basic definitions for these terms are.

Guilt: having committed an offense consciously; being worthy of blame.

Shame: painful emotion caused by consciousness of guilt or shortcoming; humiliated disgrace.

Blame: an expression of disappointment; to hold responsibility for; criticize.

What is the common theme of these definitions?

Is the source of these emotions internal or external?

Is it possible for any person to fulfill the expectations of everyone with which they interact?

When you have acted, responded to life or people in the **best** possible way that you knew how—at that point in your life's journey—what was consciously wrong about it?

Your best is all you can ask of yourself until you learn more and can do better next time.

Quick Fix

Interrupting the Guilt-Shame-Blame Cycle
Lesson 1

Make meaning for life and your actions using your spiritual nature and intuition as guides. Identify the lessons learned from your mistakes versus self-defeating dialog.

Build a bridge from your head to your heart. Create choices that nurture your core values, and are congruent with your needs, feelings, thoughts, and behavior.

Sustain this inner congruency by "walking your talk." Explore ways to give your prayers feet, and to live your heart's language.

Establish a balance of energy in with energy out. Recognize that overcaring can bleed you of energy and drain your immune system.

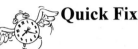 **Quick Fix**

Interrupting the Guilt-Shame-Blame Cycle
Lesson 2

Healing Interventions	Healthy Emotional Replacements
Validate and honor feelings to decrease denial of your needs.	Replace guilt with self-trust and respect.
Identify your positive attributes and contributions.	Replace shame with healthy ownership and realize that toxic shame is usually learned.
Begin to set limits and define what behavior is not comfortable or acceptable for you.	Replace *blame* with ***becoming** the best person I can be*.

Use assertions like:
*I am **comfortable** with this situation.*
*I cannot **accept** this behavior.*
*I can **tolerate** this decision.*

Choose friends and family
based on earned respect,
trust, and interdependency
versus co-dependency and
the vicious guilt-shame -
blame cycle.

Remember that if you feel
halfhearted about anything,
it usually means that you're
in the wrong place.

Create *choices* and alternatives for future actions,
change, and behavior.

Take responsibility for your
own behavior.

———————————————————

Healing boundaries means to reclaim your*self*, a
process of discovering all that is powerful and lovable
within you. Can you think of a healthier method to travel
through life than to develop a viable *container* in which to
travel? Our physical bodies provide the muscles for loco-
motion, and yet many people confuse boundary issues with
their body image. These persons add girth to create increased personal space, and may not be addressing their
very need to heal or establish boundaries that sustain total
well-being and health. Once an individual feels *safe*,

empowered as their own guardian and keeper, discriminating, and supported, there is less of a need to hide what they need and feel. Methods of hiding, especially when one is without healthy boundaries, are isolation, withdrawal, sleep, addictions, and vocations that allow their human contacts to be superficial, brief, and low-risk. Please use any of these assessment measures to increase your own level of self-discovery, and to identify where or if you need assistance or counseling with this process.

Spirituality

Spirituality is an inner light, a guiding beacon for our life journey. Develop trust and honor your intuition as a valid internal mentor. One's intuition as the language of the soul can become a travel companion of spirituality. Spirituality is the essential goodness that resides within your heart and reflects in your thoughts and actions. The idea of spirituality is often confused with religion, and it is important to recognize them as not being synonymous. Religion is an artificial construct, highly structured, external, and allows an individual to be a passive-recipient.

Spirituality is a birthright bestowed upon us by our Creator from the very beginning. Healthy spirituality is based on quality and viewing each other as a reflection of God's love. It allows us to feel pride in our very being. Guilt, shame, and fear are largely a residual of unhealthy religion in which fear of God is the major motivator versus love and forgiveness.

Journal

Where do you feel most spiritually connected?

What is your definition of spirituality?

How do you talk with your Creator?

What lesson have you learned from your religious experiences?

Imagine how different our society and we as individuals would be if from the very beginning we embraced the concept that God is forever with us, that we'd never be alone, that prayer was dialog from our heart with God, and that sometimes we need to be very quiet and *listen* for His reply.

What would be different if we learned that His forgiveness and love were unconditional and that any human offense would be forgiven if only we asked for it? What if we learned that, when we understand the least and are angry at the world, we often slam the door on God and blame Him for the trails of life. I believe that often God puts us flat on our back so that we are forced to look up or to slow down long enough to readjust our priorities.

Spirituality is living networking. It connects every living thing and provides a profound sense of belonging and grace. T.S. Eliot wrote, "Tell me what kind of God you believe in and I'll tell you what kind of person you are."

Appendix A

Self-Concept Reprogramming Model

The following model was my visual conception at the end of my master's thesis on Self-Concept Reprogramming. Because I am a visual learner, and suspect that many of you may be as well, I've chosen to include it as a summary. The following dynamic model identifies the external variables which impact our self-validation and challenges to adapt. The arrows on the model represent a two-way action with stress as a catalyst. Self-concept is the nucleus of this interacting, evolving, growing dynamic human system. The merging of the shaded areas surrounding the nucleus depicts the capacity of one's self-concept to contract and expand. Alterations in one's self-concept would result from his perceptions, behavior, aspirations, and the impact of the other designated variables.

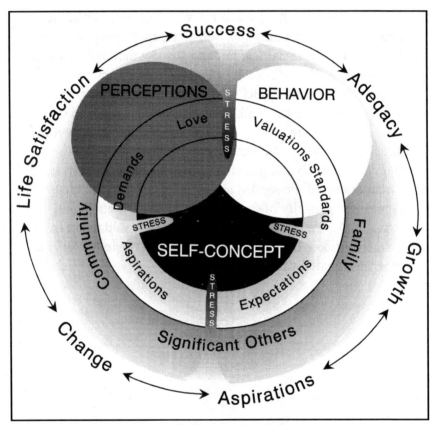

Self-Concept Model

Appendix B

Facts about B-Complex Vitamins

1. The most important thing to remember is that **all** B vitamins should be taken together in **complex** form.

2. B-Complex consists of thiamine, riboflavin, pyridoxine, B12, niacin, pantothenic acid, choline, inositol, biotin, PABA, pangamic acid (B15), and folic acid.

3. B vitamins are water soluble.

4. The more foods you eat, the more B vitamins you need.

5. Synthetic vitamin B preparations do not supply you with the same effective B-complex you get from natural sources.

6. B-complex is chiefly responsible for the health of the digestive tract, the skin, mouth, tongue, eyes, nerves, arteries, and liver.

7. Certain B vitamins redistribute body fat; Vitamin B converts fats into energy.

8. B vitamins are necessary for normal functioning of the nervous system.

9. Infection and stress increase need for B-complex.

10. B vitamins help to produce productive antibodies.

11. B vitamins may also help these ailments: beriberi, pellagra, constipation, burning feet, tender gums, burning and drying eyes, fatigue, lack of appetite, skin disorders, cracks at the corner of the mouth, and anemia.

12. Adequate amount of B-complex have been found to control migraine headaches and attacks of Meniere's Syndrome.

13. Massive dosages have been used to cure polio, improve cases of shingles, and post-operative nausea and vomiting (resulting from anesthesia).

14. One reason there is so much B vitamin deficiencies in the American population is that Americans eat so much processed foods from which the B vitamins have been removed or destroyed.

15. B vitamins help maintain elasticity in heart and digestive tract.

16. B vitamin destroyers
    a. Intense heat
    b. Slow cooking
    c. Light
    d. Baking soda
    e. Baking powder
    f. Sulfa drugs
    g. Sleeping pills
    h. Estrogen
    i. Coffee
    j. Alcohol
    k. Sugar
    l. Preservatives
    m. Florescent lighting

Glossary

Affectual reality- the status of our emotional and feeling world, both internal and external

Affect- 1) a person's emotional feeling tone. Affect and emotion are commonly used interchangeably. 2) the emotional reactions associated with an experience. syn: psychic trauma.

Affectual- feeling or emotion, the conscious, subjective aspect of an emotion considered apart from bodily changes

Assertive- to state or express positively; boldly positive

Assertiveness- any structured situation that eases the acquisition of emotionally expressive behavior; taking ownership for what we need and how to express these needs

Centering-to center or bring the mind/body back into balance; to focus or concentrate our energy forces within our biological center.

Cognitive- the process by which we decode information presented by a sensory inlet. This decoding process depends very heavily on the individual's frame of reference, sense of self, and memory. This informational process is a result of sensory and brain cortical decoding.

Cognition- level of awareness, having perception and memory skills.

Consistently conserving- 1) strategies that save energy with steady regularity and harmonious continuity; 2) showing steady conformity to a conserving character, belief, or custom; 3) to be *persistent* at saving your human resources

Corporate mentality- residual mindset especially of the subjects within the corporate jurisdiction; the byproduct of corporatism

Corporatism- the organization of a society into industrial and professional corporations, which serve as political representatives and exercising control over persons and activities under

149

their jurisdiction

Cross-brain- activities which integrate the right and left hemisphere of one's brain. Under stress, the left hemisphere tends to dominate resulting in increased verbal and intellectual struggle. This struggle can be within themselves or their environment. Centering and cross-brain balancing allows individuals to access the right hemisphere and gain greater creative, intuitive, and aesthetic resources. This will result in more holistic problem solving and effective coping with everyday stressors.

Emotive- of or relating to emotions, appealing or expressing emotion; the language of emotions

Emotive violation- 1) an infringement or transgression of one's emotional expression; 2) an act of irreverence or to rape one of their emotional integrity

Evaluative- to determine the value, significance, worth after careful appraisal and study.

Free word association- spontaneous, uncensored verbalization of whatever words come to mind

Metaphors- when a word or phrase literally denotes or elicits the idea or emotional/spiritual response; 2) to transfer the experience using a cue word or phrase

Micromanagement- to manage by focusing on only one part instead of the organizational whole

Mirroring- to reflect back

Orgasm- a peak sensory experience; a state of paroxysmal emotional excitement

Peristalsis- a wavelike, progressive movement which occurs involuntarily in hollow tubes of the body, e.g., digestive tract; 2) the wave like motion which results from simultaneous contraction and relaxation of circular muscles; 3) moving the contents forward in a spiral fashion

Projection- a defense mechanism whereby that which is emotionally unacceptable in the self is rejected and attributed to others

Subordinacy- 1) the act or position of being submissive or inferior to another person or event; 2) allowing oneself to be controlled or subservient to another influence or variable

TMJ- Tempromandiblar joint; the joint which attaches the lower jaw to the skull.

"Walking your talk"- 1) centered role-modeling; 2) operationalize our beliefs, give mobility to our core values; 3) actualize our inner truths

References

Bland, J. (1987) *Assess Your Own Nutrient Status*. Self-Care Library. New Canaan, CT: Keats.

Bland, J. (1987) *Evaluate Your Own Biochemical Individuality. Self-Care Library*. New Canaan, CT: Keats.

Booth, L. (1992) *When God Becomes a Drug: Understanding Religious Addiction & Religious Abuse*. New York: Putnam.

Chopra, Deepak. (1991) *Perfect Health*. New York: Harmony Books.

Kunin, R. (1982) *Mega-Nutrition*. New York: Mosby.

Caine, R.N. & Caine, G. (1991) *Making Connections: Teaching and the Human Brain*. Alexandria, VA: Association for Supervision and Curriculum Development.

Fortuna, J. (1992) *Food for Recovery*. (video recording) Denver, CO: MAC Publishing.

Garrison, R.H. & Womer, E. (1985) *The Nutrition Desk Reference*. New Canaan: Keats.

Guyton, A.C. (1976) *Textbook of Medical Physiology. Fifth Edition*. Philadelphia: W.B. Saunders.

Kellogg, T.& Harrison, M. (1991) *Finding Balance: Twelve Priorities for Interdependence & Joyful Living*. Deerfield Beach, FL: Health Communications.

Lerner, R. (1990) *Affirmations for the Inner Child*. Deerfield Beach, FL: Health Communications.

Samuels, M. and Samuels, N. (1975) *Seeing with the Mind's Eye: The History, Techniques and Uses of Visualization*. New York: Random House.

Walz, J. (1979) *Effects on Self-Concept after Participation in a Six-Week Course on Self-Awareness, Perception, & Stress Management*. Unpublished master's thesis. Marquette University, Milwaukee, WI.

Index

1:2 breathing sequence 104

accountability 50
adrenal gland 70, 76, 77
affectual reality 23, 149
affirmations 30, 40, 105, 111,
              130, 133
anger 11, 18, 24, 54, 63, 123
antioxidants 77, 78
assertiveness 47
attention deficit disorder 59,
              81
attributes 29, 30, 34, 139

baroreceptors 100
beta carotene 69, 77, 78, 147
blood glucose 59
body image 15, 21, 34-37, 140
boundaries 20, 39-40, 119,
              127-141
boundary affirmations 130

calcium 66-68, 72, 76, 147
capillary-alveolar unit 102
cardiovascular 70
center 22, 46, 53, 110, 122,
              129, 149
centered role-modeling 27,
              151
color 94, 109
components of self-concept 15,
              21
consistent 29, 98, 129, 130

constructive 11, 26, 30, 36,
              105, 120, 129,
              134
core values 16, 31-32, 48, 52,
              131, 138, 151
corner stones 123
cortisol 76, 84
creativity 16, 89, 90-95, 107
cross brain 106

deep breathing 72
defense mechanisms 132, 134
downshifting 54
dynamic model 143

effective problem solving 27
elastin 71
emotive violation 130, 150
epitaph 31
external control center 16

facts 18, 25, 27, 41, 53
fair 29, 129
fat-soluble vitamins 71
free word association 121, 128,
              150

gastrointestinal system 74
genetic legacy 62, 63

hiding 141
humor 30, 107, 108
hypoglycemia 59, 68
hypoxia 101

153

tryptophane 79
tyramine 80-81
tyrosine 79

unlearning 34, 120

validations 29
visual imagery 108, 110, 111
vitamin A 69, 77, 147
vitamin B complex 64-65, 68,
            74-76, 147
vitamin E 71, 77-78, 147

warrior macrophages 76
water 70-77

zinc 69, 77, 147

Ordering Information

Quick Fixes to Change Your Life : Making Healthy Choices by Judy Walz
Order additional copies at $10.95 each + $3.00 shipping for the first book. Shipping is $1.00 for each additional book.

Breast Cancer: A Patient Guide by Patricia J. Anderson
Widely regarded as the most comprehensive "how-to" manual, this book is essential for women who have breast cancer. $14.95 + $3.00 shipping for the first book. Shipping is $1.00 for each additional book.

Breast Cancer News: Information for Survivors
Patricia J. Anderson, editor
This monthly newsletter keeps women up-to-date on the latest breast cancer information and tips for dealing with the emotional and physical side effects. $24.00/year (12 issues).

Sales Tax:
Please add local sales tax for books shipped to Georgia or Kansas.

Discounts:
Contact CHS for discounts on more than five copies shipped to the same address.

Guarantee:
Your money will be refunded if you are not satisfied.

☎ **Telephone Orders:** Call 0-700-740-6192. Have your VISA or MasterCard Ready.

* **FAX orders:** Send the order information and VISA or MasterCard number, expiration date, and name on card to (706) 568-9007.

✉ **Mail orders:** Send shipping information and payment to Creative Health Services, Inc. 7222 Westport Court, Midland, GA 31820-9040